Advanced Personal Training

A Practical Guide to Working with
Healthy & Special Needs Clients

Joe Cannon, MS

ISBN:0692293531

Printed in the United States of America

Published September 2014

TABLE of CONTENTS

CHAPTER 1
Energy Systems

Energy is the ability to do work. For example, walking and lifting weights are work and require energy. We make energy from the macronutrients we eat - carbohydrates, fats and to a lesser extent, proteins because food has energy (calories). However, before this can happen, we must transform the food energy (calories), into a form of energy that we know how to use. For humans, this energy molecule is called *adenosine triphosphate* (ATP). Think about how a car works. Cars do not run on oil. The oil has to be refined into gasoline first. We work like that too. We take the raw materials in food and refine them into a special type of *gasoline - ATP*.

The Macronutrients

Food	Calories / Gram
Protein	4
Carbohydrate	4
Fat	9

There are 28 grams in one ounce.

How Do We Make ATP?

Basically, we have two ways of making ATP. One way uses oxygen to make energy and is called the aerobic energy system. The other way does not need oxygen to work. It is called the *anaerobic energy system*. The aerobic energy system, tends to burn fat and works more at lower intensities of activity while the anaerobic system, mostly burns carbohydrates (carbs) and works at higher intensities. It's important to remember that both aerobic and anaerobic systems are always working inside of us. In other words, we are never only burning fat and we are never only burning carbs. Rather, we are, for the most part, always burning a mixture of fats and carbs to power our energy needs. At lower intensities of activity, we tend to burn greater percentages of fat, while at higher intensities of activity, we tend to burn greater percentages of carbs.

In addition, it is not only the *intensity* of activity that dictates what we burn for fuel but also the *length of time* that we can do the activity. In other words, if you can perform an activity for a long time, you are burning a large percentage of energy from fat. If you can only do the activity for a short period of time, carbohydrates (e.g., glucose) are supplying the bulk of your energy.

The Aerobic Energy System

Another name for the aerobic system is the *Krebs cycle*. The Krebs cycle is a complex series of chemical reactions that essentially results in energy (ATP) being produced from the breakdown of fat. This is why people who are trying to lose weight often do aerobic activity —because the Krebs cycle uses oxygen to burn fat. The Krebs cycle occurs within the *mitochondria*, which is where fat burning occurs. Aerobic exercise training causes the mitochondria of muscles to enlarge and become more numerous. Bigger, more numerous mitochondria can burn more fat. So we would expect to see bigger and more numerous mitochondria in the muscles of a triathlete, cyclist or bodybuilder. Those not accustomed to exercise exhaust themselves quickly. One reason for this is that their mitochondria are smaller and less numerous. Thus, they are not good at fat burning. Here, their bodies rely more heavily on burning carbs (glycogen and glucose) anaerobically. This results in the build up of lactic acid that contributes to the burning sensation inside muscles that forces the person to cease exercise. Aerobically trained muscles, on the other hand, use more fat and less carbs during exercise. Since the depletion of carbs can greatly reduce exercise ability, this means that exercise-trained muscles can work longer because of their lower reliance on carbs and greater reliance on fat.

In some older adults artery-clogging plaque builds within the blood vessels of the legs and reduces oxygen delivery to the muscles. This ramps up lactic acid production and causes the person to experience calf and leg pain quickly after they start to walk. When they sit down, the pain goes away. Fitness trainers should be aware of this because it may be a sign of heart disease - specifically peripheral artery disease (PAD). This is a serious medical disorder. Those with PAD should inform their physician before starting an exercise program. After medical clearance, these individuals are better suited by aerobic exercise on a bike or in a pool rather than exercise that requires them to stand.

The Anaerobic Energy System

The anaerobic energy system basically has two parts: the *ATP/CP system* and *glycolysis*. The ATP/CP system (adenosine triphosphate /creatine phosphate) is sometimes called the *phosphagen system* because phosphate is found in both compounds. When exercise is very intense, creatine phosphate is activated. Creatine Phosphate (or phosphocreatine) is used to replenish ATP faster than all other aerobic and anaerobic systems. This is why people often take creatine supplements. Remember that CP itself cannot provide energy. Only by helping reenergize ATP is CP able to contribute to our energy needs. Generally, our cells can store four to six times more CP than ATP. This extra energy boost from CP can provide about an extra 10-20 seconds of activity during high intensity exercise.[1]

Creatine is not used significantly during low intensity activities like walking, hiking or circuit weight-training. For more information on creatine and more than 100 other supplements, read *Nutritional Supplements: What Works and Why,* available at www.Joe-Cannon.com.

The other part of the anaerobic system is called *glycolysis*. Glycolysis refers to a series of chemical reactions in which ATP (energy) is made via the anaerobic breakdown of carbs. Glycolysis is also sometimes called the *lactic acid system* because *lactic acid* a is formed during glycolysis. The fuel of choice used in glycolysis is glucose. Glucose is a simple sugar the body prefers to use and is the reason it is often called "blood sugar." In fact, some organs of the body (e.g., the brain) must have glucose to function. If the body cannot use glucose, diabetes results.

Some say that lactic acid is a waste product. This is not true. For example, growth hormone release appears to be tied to lactic acid production.

CHAPTER 2
Anatomy For Personal Trainers

Muscle tissue can be divided into three types: smooth muscle, cardiac muscle and skeletal muscle. *Smooth muscle* lines blood vessels and allows them to expand and contract when needed. *Cardiac muscle* is heart muscle. *Skeletal muscle* is the type that is usually of most interest to fitness professionals. It is called skeletal muscle because, for the most part, it is attached to the skeleton (e.g., biceps.).

Connective tissue refers to a diverse type of tissues that serve many different functions. Blood, bone, tendons and cartilage are all examples of connective tissues. Cartilage helps form joints, ribs, tendons, ligaments and ears. Because of its dense nature, cartilage is able to sustain great forces without being damaged. This makes cartilage perfect for the ends of the long bones of the body (e.g. femur) where it helps reduce friction and absorb shocks. During the disorder, osteoarthritis (OA) this cartilage is damaged resulting in pain as bones grind together. Cartilage has no direct blood supply. This is why tendons and ligaments take so long to heal after they are injured.

A tendon is a tough band of connective tissue that usually connects muscles to bones. This is why it's possible for strength training to build bones and help osteoporosis. In other words, as you strengthen muscles you also strengthen bones. At the point where the tendon and muscle come together is a specialized sensor called the *Golgi tendon organ* (GTO). The GTO monitors force production by the muscle. If the GTO senses that the muscle may be injured by too much force the GTO activates. When this happens, the GTO relaxes the muscle! In extreme instances, the GTO may also cause the contraction of the opposing muscle to further help reduce injury! You can think of the GTO as a safety mechanism that protects the body from harm. But, consider the person who lifts so much weight that the GTO activates. The GTO "thinks" that an injury is about to occur. It doesn't "know" that the person has 300 pounds suspended above his/her body! This is why lifters should always have a spotter.

Ligaments are also made of connective tissue and connect the bones together. When one bone is connected to another, a *joint* is formed. There are 206 bones in the adult human body. Bones act as a reservoir for minerals (e.g., calcium) if needed. There are four types of bones in the body: long bones, short bones, flat bones and irregularly- shaped bones. The bone shaft of long bones is called the *diaphysis* and the ends of these bones are called the *epiphysis*. It is at the ends of long bones (epiphysis) that bones grow longer. These regions are called the *epithelial plates* (growth plates). Damage to growth plates is often cited as a reason to deter children from lifting weights. While possible, research also finds that supervised resistance training can also help reduce injuries in adolescents.[2]

Bone growth and repair is complex; however, three types of cells are usually described. They are osteoblasts, osteocytes and osteoclasts. *Osteoblasts* are immature bone cells. Osteoblast cells eventually become mature bone cells called osteocytes. Osteoclasts are bone-eating cells. As osteoclasts degrade bone, minerals (e.g., calcium) are released for the body to use if adequate nutrients are not consumed in the diet. Ultimately, this process can lead to bone being degraded faster than it can be made, resulting in a loss of bone density and ultimately osteoporosis. Fortunately, because muscles are attached to the bones it is possible for strength training to improve osteoporosis. It's important for fitness professionals to remember that osteoporosis is not simply a condition that affects people who are "old." Long-term bed rest, various diseases or just not moving enough can all lead to reduced bone density. Men get osteoporosis too. Some evidence hints that the greatest rate of bone loss occurs within the first seven weeks of no physical activity.[3]

Human Skeleton Front View

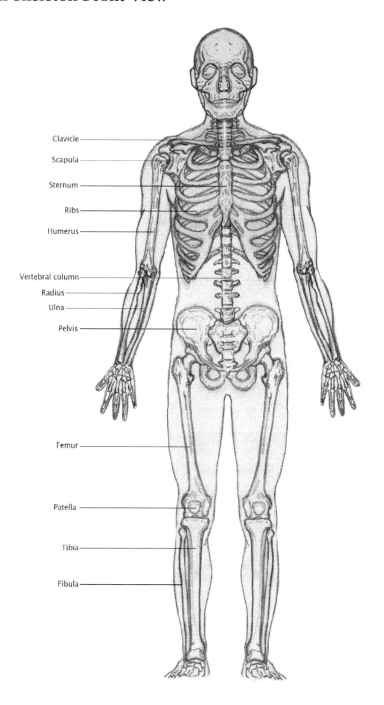

Clavicle

Scapula

Sternum

Ribs

Humerus

Vertebral column

Radius

Ulna

Pelvis

Femur

Patella

Tibia

Fibula

Human Skeleton. Back View

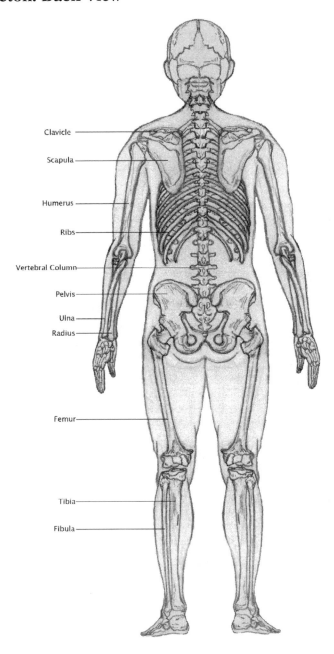

Clavicle

Scapula

Humerus

Ribs

Vertebral Column

Pelvis

Ulna

Radius

Femur

Tibia

Fibula

CHAPTER 3
Muscle Physiology For Personal Trainers

Muscles are made of muscle fibers, also called muscle cells. If you could pull one of your muscle cells out of your body and look deep inside you would see that the fiber is made up of even smaller units called myofibrils.[4] Myofibrils, are composed of a variety of myofilament proteins. Two of these proteins are myosin and actin. *Myosin* is a thick protein. *Actin* is a thinner protein. These myosin and actin proteins are layered or stacked on top of one another inside myofibrils and make up the force generating functional unit of muscle contraction called a *sarcomere*. When a muscle contracts, it is the sarcomeres which make up that muscle fiber that actually contract. Muscles are able to contract because the actin and myosin proteins slide over each other. The process that explains how this happens is known as the Sliding Filament Theory.

Types of Muscle Fibers

Many have heard that we have slow twitch and fast twitch muscle fibers. But there is another naming system that fitness trainers often use that is better. This is because there is more than one type of fast twitch fiber. We often call slow twitch *type I fibers* and fast twitch *type II fibers*. Type II fibers can be further divided into type IIa and type IIb muscle fibers.

Type I muscle fibers are small fibers that produce low amounts of force, but they can produce that force for long periods of time. Thus, type I fibers are hard to fatigue. This is because they are aerobic fibers that contain an abundance mitochondria and capillaries which allow them to burn fat and glucose for energy. They are purely aerobic fibers and generally do not have the ability to work anaerobically. They are called type I because they are usually the first muscle fibers that are activated when a muscle contracts.

Type IIa muscle fibers can make energy both aerobically and anaerobically because they use glycolysis, the Krebs cycle and the ATP/CP energy systems. In other words, they can burn fat, carbs and creatine. These are usually the second type of fiber that is recruited into action.

Type IIb fibers are the most powerful fibers in the body. As such, they are used during activities that are perceived as very demanding such as powerlifting, sprinting, etc. But, the power they produce doesn't last long. Thus, type IIb fibers are also the quickest to fatigue.[5] Two reasons for this is that they have the lowest number of mitochondria and capillaries (both of which are needed to burn fat). Type IIb fibers are strictly anaerobic and so only use glycolysis and the APT/CP system to generate energy. In other words, they burn glucose and creatine only. These are often the third (or last) fiber to be recruited.

Quick Reference

Muscle Fiber Type	Brief Description
Skeletal muscle	Mostly attached to skeleton. Also called voluntary muscle.
Type I muscle fibers	Aerobic only. Endurance fibers. Use fat and carbs.
Type IIa muscle fibers	Both aerobic & anaerobic. Strength & endurance fibers.
Type IIb muscle fibers	Anaerobic only. Powerful fibers. Fatigue very fast.

Muscle Fibers Types

Commonly used name	Commonly used name	Scientific name
Type I fibers	Slow twitch	Slow Oxidative fibers (SO fibers)
Type IIa fibers	Fast twitch	Fast oxidative glycolytic fibers (FOG fibers)
Type IIb fibers	Fast twitch	Fast Glycolytic fibers (FG fibers)

Can exercise can change muscle fiber type? Technically this cannot happen however it is possible to change the internal make-up of a muscle fiber by training. For example, research suggests that, with exercise, type IIb fibers begin to take on characteristics of type IIa fibers.[6] This may be because type IIa fibers are more useful than type IIb in that they are almost as powerful and can do a lot of things type IIb can't. That doesn't mean type IIb fibers are useless. Many activities require power and personal trainers may have need to develop these fibers in some clients. Type I fibers might also start to "look" like type IIa fibers when the correct type of exercise is performed. Humans don't seem to be able make a type I fiber act like a type IIb or vice versa.

Hypertrophy, Hyperplasia and Atrophy

Hypertrophy refers to an increase in the size of a muscle and is the main way muscles increase in strength. Basically, exercise increases the production of muscle proteins. The more muscle proteins in a muscle fiber the bigger it gets and more force it can develop. If exercise training stops, muscles eventually lose strength (and size) resulting in atrophy. Generally, atrophy becomes significant 2-3 weeks after exercise stops. With constant bed rest, significant atrophy may occur after one week. Anything that limits movement -obesity, heart disease etc - causes atrophy.

Hyperplasia refers to the growth of new muscle fibers. Whether or not humans can grow new fibers is controversial although in theory, it may be possible. If hyperplasia occurs in humans, it's probably only a minor contributor for most healthy people.

Sarcopenia refers to loss of muscle mass and strength during the aging process. Normally sarcopenia starts in the 30s-40s. After 50, sarcopenia accelerates. The result is a loss of not only strength but independence, causing many to enter nursing homes. Lack of muscle strength means people will move less (including exercise). This in turn increases the risk of heart disease, diabetes, cancer and many other conditions. Sarcopenia destroys all muscle fibers however it is type II fibers that are mostly impacted. Both men and women get sarcopenia; however, some research hints that men may experience sarcopenia to a greater degree than women. But, because women outlive men, they may live with the ravages of sarcopenia for a longer time. Genetics certainly plays a role in sarcopenia. However, it's also true that lack of proper exercise and nutrition contribute. Fitness trainers more than any other member of the health care system can educate people about sarcopenia and reduce its impact. It's ironic that very few people - including fitness trainers - have ever heard of a condition that effects everybody.

Types of Muscle Actions

There are three different types of muscle actions (muscle contractions). They are isometric muscle actions, isokinetic muscle actions and isotonic (dynamic) muscle actions. Of these, human muscles usually perform either isometric actions or the more frequently occurring, isotonic muscle actions.

Isotonic (Dynamic) Muscle Actions

This is the type of muscle actions we do most. The term isotonic refers to constant tension being produced inside the muscle and how the muscle length changes as we go through a movement's safe range of motion (ROM). Isotonic muscle actions are composed of two phases – concentric and eccentric. Concentric muscle actions occur when we are lifting the weight. If we could look at the muscle cell during a concentric muscle action, we would see that it is shortening as force is applied. Eccentric muscle actions (*negatives*) usually occur when we are lowering a weight. During eccentric actions, the actin and myosin proteins are being pulled apart. This causes the muscle to lengthen as force is applied to it.

Eccentric muscle actions can result in greater improvements of strength and higher metabolic rates compared to concentric movements. The downside is that eccentrics also result in a more delayed onset muscle soreness (DOMS).[7]

Isometric Muscle Actions

Isometric muscle actions occur when no change in muscle length occurs as the muscle is used. Another name that refers to isometrics is static contractions. Isometrics will increase muscle strength; but they are less effective than isotonic muscle actions. Isometrics also raise blood pressure more than other modes of strength training.[8] As such, they are not recommended for people with high blood pressure or heart disease.

Isokinetic Muscle Actions

Isokinetic muscle actions occur at the same speed throughout the range of motion. This is not a real-life movement because when we exercise, our muscles do not move at the same speed. To do isokinetic movements you need special equipment.

Delayed Onset Muscle Soreness

Delayed onset muscle soreness (DOMS) is muscle pain felt after a strenuous or unaccustomed activity. The pain often occurs 24 to 72 hours after exercise and subsides 7 to 10 days later. Anything that's intense enough or that you are not used to doing will cause DOMS if you do it long enough. During this time, people may not be able to lift as much. This is because of both a decreased ability of the muscle to produce force and persons unwillingness to use the muscles.[9] DOMS does result in short-term muscle damage.[10]

There are several theories to explain DOMS. But, no single theory fully explains the process. Regardless of what causes DOMS, what we do know is that eccentric activities or "negatives" cause more DOMS than concentric movements.[11]

DOMS Myth Busting

Does lactic acid build up cause DOMS? There is no proof of this. Lactic acid is normally cleared from muscles within 1-2 hrs after exercise.

Can stretching help? There is not much evidence that stretching sore muscles alleviates DOMS. Likewise stretching before exercise does not seem to reduce DOMS either. In fact, evidence suggests that stretching can *cause* DOMS, if you are not used to stretching.[12] Stretching between sets however may speed recovery during subsequent sets. Also, using antioxidant supplements to protect against DOMS or speed relief has is not fully accepted.[13] Do sports creams help? These mask pain with sensations of heat or cold but do not speed recovery from DOMS. Currently, the only accepted therapy for reducing DOMS is performing a low intensity set of the exercise a day or two before the actual workout.[14]

DOMS is not felt when the muscle is not moving. We only feel DOMS when the muscles are moved or when they are touched.[15] This can sometimes help fitness trainers differentiate between DOMS and other more serious types of pain.

Rhabdomyolysis

Rhabdomyolysis is a very serious condition all fitness trainers should be aware of. It is possible to die from rhabdomyolysis.[16] This is a condition where muscle cells rupture from an overwhelming stress. Exercise-induced rhabdomyolysis results when exercise overwhelms the body's ability to adapt. This can result after a single workout.[17] Rhabdomyolysis has been reported in soldiers, firemen, law enforcement trainees, football players, bodybuilders and marathoners.[18] Activities that focus on eccentric muscle actions appear to increase its incidence. At least one case report has shown rhabdomyolysis resulting from overzealous personal trainers.[19] Classic signs of this condition include kidney failure, heart attack and intense muscle soreness and weakness. The pain felt with this condition happens faster than with DOMS (e.g. within 24 hrs). Another sign is very dark-colored urine.[18] This means blood in the urine. How much exercise will cause rhabdomyolysis? This is likely different for everybody. In one report, a 29-year-old man developed rhabdomyolysis after performing 30 sit-ups a day for 5 days.[20] Fitness trainers who conduct hard-core or boot-camp type workouts must always be aware of rhabdomyolysis when they conduct exercise sessions.

CHAPTER 4
Cardiovascular Physiology For Personal Trainers

The cardiovascular system is composed primarily of the heart, blood, blood vessels and lungs as well as muscles, tissues and chemical pathways that help support the absorption and transport of oxygen and nutrients through the blood and removal of waste products that build up during exercise and as a natural consequence of being alive. Blood contains red blood cells (RBCs) that carry oxygen. They are able to do this because RBCs contain hemoglobin that gives blood its red color. Blood travels through vessels called arteries and veins. Arteries carry blood away from the heart. As blood travels from the heart, the arteries get smaller and become capillaries. It is in the capillaries that oxygen and other nutrients are exchanged for waste products. From here, veins carry blood back to the heart. Blood vessels are not simply hose-like tubes. Rather, they expand and contract. Some may have heard of the amino acid arginine which helps make nitric oxide (NO). Nitric oxide expands blood vessels. Most of these supplements need more study and may carry some risks.[13] Fitness trainers should be able to sort fact from fiction about supplements.

Each day the heart pumps about 2000 gallons of blood. The pumping of blood is facilitated by the hearts chambers. The heart has 4 chambers - 2 atria and 2 ventricles.

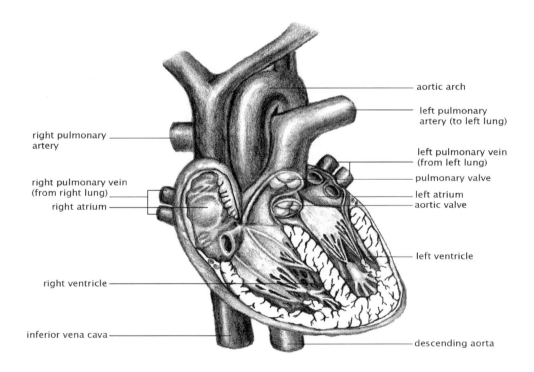

Blood first enters the heart at the right atria and leaves the heart (to be pumped throughout the body) from the left ventricle. The left ventricle heart muscle is strong and is the reason why when it contracts, it pushes the blood from the heart. Because it is a muscle, the heart gets stronger when we exercise (especially aerobic exercise) and the muscle in the left ventricle gets stronger too. Stronger left ventricle heart muscles means a greater contraction force to push blood from the heart. The better the heart can pump blood the better our aerobic fitness. Doctors often measure three aspects of heart fitness: stroke volume, ejection fraction and cardiac output.

Stroke volume is the amount of blood pumped from the heart (left ventricle) in a heartbeat. As the heart gets stronger, stroke volume improves. The ejection fraction measures how much blood was ejected from the heart compared to the volume in the heart *before* the heart contracted. If you had one pint of blood in your heart and the heart ejected 60% of that point, your ejection fraction is 60%. Ejection fraction improves with exercise training also. Cardiac output is the total output of blood from your heart in one minute. It also improves when we exercise regularly. The result of all of this is the heart can deliver more blood to the muscles and cells of the body and remove waste products faster. This means our aerobic fitness is improved. Many other positive outcomes are seen with long-term aerobic (CV) exercise as well.

Benefits of Chronic Aerobic Exercise

↑stroke volume	↑ejection fraction	↑cardiac output	↓RHR	↓LDL	↑HDL
↓total cholesterol	↓blood pressure	↑capillary density	↓CAD	↓ HTN	↓ cancer
↑ antioxidants	↑ immunity	↑ RBCs	↑ fat oxidation	↓ triglycerides	↓ risk of death

Partial list of benefits. CAD=heart disease. HTN = hypertension. RHR = resting heart rate.

Resting heart rate (RHR) is often used as a measure of fitness. An average, healthy RHR can range from 60-100bpm. Those who exercise regularly may have an RHR of 40bpm! However, be cautious of a low RHR in someone who does not exercise. This may indicate the person takes drugs for high blood pressure.

Moderate exercise training can improve the immune system.[21] Exhaustive exercise (a marathon), however, can reduce immunity.[22] Exercise can reduce total cholesterol and "bad" cholesterol (LDL) as well as raise "good" cholesterol (HDL).[23] Triglycerides can also lower with exercise.[23] These, help lower risk of heart disease (CAD), the number one killer of Americans.

Heart Disease Risk Factors

Family History	Heart attack, heart disease surgery or sudden death before the age of 55 in father or immediate relative (son, brother) or before the age of 65 in mother or other immediate relative (sister, daughter)
Smoking	Someone who is a current smoker or one who quit smoking in the last 6 months
High Blood Pressure	Blood pressure > 140/90 mm Hg or on medications for high blood pressure
High Cholesterol	Total cholesterol > 200 mg/dl or HDL < 40 mg /dl or someone taking medications for high cholesterol. Someone whose LDL cholesterol is > 100 mg/dl
Obesity	BMI > 30 kg/m^2 or having a waist circumference > 100 cm
Sedentary	Not doing at least 30 minutes of sustained activity most days of the week

An HDL of 60 or better is a "negative risk factor" for heart disease. This lowers the risk of heart disease.

Exercising to exhaustion is also not warranted in those with immune system problems such as HIV/AIDS. Likewise exhaustive exercise should not be performed in those with joint disorders like rheumatoid arthritis because it can lead to greater rates of injury. In diabetics, intense exercise might raise blood sugar levels to dangerous levels while working out to exhaustion might lower blood sugar too much.

Much research shows that exercise improves the body's natural antioxidant defenses. Antioxidants neutralize compounds called free radicals which can cause disease. Many people think that antioxidants only come from supplements. They don't know that we have natural antioxidants that help protect us from free radicals. This may be one of the reasons that exercise helps protect against diseases like cancer.

The amount of exercise to achieve all of the benefits of exercise can vary. For general health 30- 60 minutes of moderate intensity exercise most days of the week is often recommended. It also appears that several, shorter exercise sessions confer the same benefit as a single longer session. For example, three 20 minute exercise sessions a day appear to be just as good as a single 60 minute workout. This is great news for people with limited time to exercise.

Blood Pressure

Blood pressure (BP) is the force of the blood, exerted against the walls of the blood vessels as blood is pumped through the body. Blood pressure as really made up of two different pressures. The *systolic pressure* is the blood pressure during the pumping phase of the heart cycle. The *diastolic pressure* is the blood pressure during the filling phase, just before the heart pumps again. Systolic pressure is the top number of the blood pressure fraction and diastolic pressure is the bottom number. So, if your BP was 125/80, the systolic BP is 125 and 80 is the diastolic BP. Many things alter blood pressure. Smoking, sodium and alcohol abuse can raise blood pressure. So too can being overweight/obese. BP tends to rise as we age as well. Exercise can raise blood pressure also but only when you are working out. When you exercise, systolic BP tends to go up as intensity is increased, while diastolic BP tends to not change. Regular exercise often lowers both systolic and diastolic BP, especially in those with high blood pressure (HTN). Many people have high blood pressure so fitness trainers should be aware of what is normal and not normal BP.

Blood Pressure Guidelines[24]

< 120/80	Normal
120/80 - 139/89	Prehypertension
≥ 140/90	Hypertension

Notice that a BP that's less than 120/80 is "normal". A reading of 120/80 is the start of "prehypertension" or pre high blood pressure. This is because of finding that in men, age 55 and older, a BP of 120/80 appears to increase the chances of future high blood pressure by 90%..[24] High blood pressure contributes to stroke, the 3rd leading cause of death in America. Fitness trainers who take BP should not diagnose a client as having hypertension. Only a doctor can do this.

CHAPTER 5
Creating an Exercise Program

Before an exercise program can be designed, the personal trainer should preferably know not only the health issues of the person but their overall current fitness level as well. Usually fitness trainers will test one or more of the following categories to estimate the overall fitness of the person:

1. **Muscular strength:** The ability of a muscle to exert force.

2. **Muscular endurance:** The ability of a muscle to contract repeatedly over time.

3. **Cardiovascular endurance:** The ability of the heart, lungs and blood vessels to deliver oxygen and nutrients to the exercising muscles and remove waste products.

4. **Flexibility:** The range of motion of a joint.

5. **Body composition:** The amount of muscle and fat present on the body.

6. **Balance**: The ability to maintain balance during every day activities.

There are many tests for each fitness category. No single test is always appropriate in all people. The trainer must use a test that is both safe for the person and relatively accurate and can be easily reproduced. A review of fitness tests can be found at the end of this chapter.

To design a safe and effective exercise program, trainers must know the basic principles of exercise.

Principle of Specificity. Exercise needs to be specific to the needs of the person and progress as the persons needs, goals and fitness improve. At the core of this is the SAID Principle. SAID stands for *specific adaptations to imposed demands.* Basically, the body will respond specifically to those exercise demands that are imposed upon it. In other words, if you want to be better at the bench press, then do the bench press. Do what you want/need to be better at, and you will improve at it.

Principle of Overload. Fitness will not improve unless the body is overloaded a little more than it is used to. Trainers overload people by altering 4 key components that are called the FITT Principle, where FITT stands for:

- Frequency of exercise. Ex. Increasing from 2 to 3 days per week
- Intensity of exercise. Ex. Increasing from 2-2.5 mph on a treadmill
- Time of exercise. Ex. Increasing from a 30 min workout to a 40 min workout
- Type of exercise. Ex. Instead of using a treadmill, use the elliptical.

Principle of Adaptation. Eventually we get used to the exercise program. To improve further, it must be changed. For example, if you always lift weights first, try doing cardio first.

Principle of Individual differences. Different people may respond differently to a program.

The Importance of The Warm Up

A general warm up is low intensity aerobic activity lasting about 5-10 minutes. This prepares the body for the harder workout ahead. Stretching is not a good warm up because most people only stretch for a few seconds. Warming up has many benefits such as[25]

1. improved reaction time
2. improved flexibility
3. increased metabolic rate
4. possible reduced injury risk
5. possible reductions in the risk of a heart attack

Multi-Joint vs. Single Joint Exercises

A multi-joint exercise uses a lot of different muscle groups at the same time. A push up is an example. Other names include core exercises and compound exercises. These movements tend to be more real-life and better mimic activates of daily living (ADLs). They also promote greater elevations in anabolic hormones. In contrast, single joint exercises (e.g. biceps curl) use less muscle.

General Resistance Exercise Training Guidelines

1. Always warm up first

2. Don't train the same muscle group more than two days in a row

3. Multi-joint exercises should be performed *before* single joint exercises

4. Perform the hardest exercises first; the easiest/simpler exercises, do last

5. Train muscles you want to emphasize the most, early into the workout

6. Train abs/back muscles after the exercises that use those muscles (to reduce injury)

7. Teach new exercises early in the workout (to reduce injury)

8. In novices, teach machine exercises before free weight exercises

9. Do free weight exercise *before* machines if both are done in the same workout

10 Cool down and/or stretch at the end of the workout

Volume of Exercise. Volume is the total amount of work done in a workout. Volume is defined as the weight x reps x sets. If you performed 1 set of a leg press at 100 lbs for 10 reps your volume is 1 x 100 x 10 = 1000 lbs. If 2 months, later you are doing 3 sets, your volume is 3 x 100 x 10 = 3000 lbs. Volume is a very important way to gauge progression and is central to the achievement to the goals we are about to discuss in this chapter.

Training Beginners

In novices, improvements in strength for the first 8-12 weeks are mostly due to improvements in how the brain communicates with the muscles. These improvements are called neurological changes. It's after this time when significant changes in muscle hypertrophy and strength start to occur. Likewise, trainers should also recognize that while muscles tend to improve strength relatively quickly, ligaments and tendons do not. This can lead to injuries if the intensity of a program is applied too fast. As such many beginners are best suited with single set programs of first few months.[26] As for intensity, workouts should be composed of light to moderate amounts of weight. If performing strength training, this equals a load they can lift between 12-20 reps. Alternately, trainers may determine a percent of repetition maximum (RM). This refers to the most weight that can be lifted safely with good form. For example, a 12 RM is a resistance that can be lifted for only 12 reps with good form. Trainers may determine an RM value in the gym and have people train at a percentage of that value (e.g. 70% of 12 RM). Another way a resistance may be chosen is to use the RPE scale (Borg Scale). For example you might ask the person how heavy a resistance feels on a scale from zero (very, very light) to 10 (very very heavy).

How many sets should be performed per exercise? The answer depends on who the client is. While several studies find multiple set programs (e.g. 3 sets per body part) better for improving strength, they can lead to greater DOMS and injuries in beginners. Some also find multiple set programs boring. For beginners who are generally healthy with no medical issues, one set of 8-12 different exercises targeting the major muscles of the body is often recommended.[25] After 2-3 months, multiple set programs can be used if desired.

What is Periodization?

Periodization is at the core of designing and updating exercise programs. Periodization refers to breaking a workout up into different parts. During each part, the weight, reps, sets, rest periods and exercise selections are altered periodically to improve fitness and reduce injury. Traditionally, workouts are easy and general and become progressively harder and more focused to what the persons goals are as their fitness improves. In periodization there are 3 main cycles: macrocycles, mesocycles and microcycles. A macrocycle represents a whole year of training. Each macrocycle is made up of several mesocycles which last from many weeks to months. Each mesocycle is made up of many microcycles which last about a week or so. Remember, the time spent in each cycle will vary according to fitness level and time it takes to progress.

Periodization also has several periods and phases, to help the trainer further focus exercise to the desired goals. Usually trainers focus on the following:

Preparatory Period. Here the person does the work needed to prepare for their goal. This is where most people stay for most of their training. Within this period are the following phases:

1. Hypertrophy Phase.   Goal. Enhance muscle hypertrophy and endurance
2. Strength Phase.   Goal. Improve muscle strength
3. Power Phase.   Goal. Improve muscular power

Remember that not all people will have a power phase. This may also increase injuries. Aside from the phases, athletes may also incorporate a "competition phase" which is when they are competing in their sport, as well as an "active rest phase", after their sport season when they are not training hard. This allows the body to rest before harder training is undertaken for the next season. Non-athletes won't have a competition phase but everybody can benefit from active rest from time to time.

Basic Guidelines for Goal Achievement

Goal: Muscle Endurance. Resistance is usually 12-15 RM (up to 20 RM) for multi-joint exercises. If determining 1RM use < 67% 1 RM. Perform 1 to 3 sets per exercise.[4] The rest periods are less than 30 seconds between sets.[4] This protocol taxes type I fibers and the aerobic energy system (Krebs cycle) the most. This protocol is also good for people high blood pressure and arthritis and is a good starting point when training beginners.

Goal: Muscle Hypertrophy. Resistance should be between 6RM-12RM for multi-joint exercise. If determining 1RM use 67% - 85% 1 RM.[4] Do 3-6 sets per exercise. Start with one exercise per body part and progress to 3-4 exercises. Rest periods are usually 30 seconds to 1.5 minutes between sets. This protocol taxes mostly aerobic and anaerobic energy systems and type I and II fibers. This is a very high volume routine so much DOMS can occur. Not for beginners.

Goal: Muscular Strength. Resistance should be between 6-10 RM for multi-joint exercises. If determining 1RM use > 85% 1 RM.[4] Perform 2-6 sets per exercise. Rest periods between sets are 2-3 minutes. This protocol works mostly type II fibers and the anaerobic (glycolysis) energy system. This also improves bone density but puts much stress on joints with arthritis. Not for beginners.

Goal: Muscular Power. Resistance should be 1-2RM for multi-joint activities or 90% - 100% 1RM. Perform 1-5 sets. Rest periods are 2-5 minutes between sets. This intensity should not be performed for single joint exercises because of high injury risk. This procedure activates type II fibers (usually all muscle fibers too) and the ATP/CP system. This also improves bone density but is not good for those with arthritis or high blood pressure. Not for beginners.

Review of Strength Training Programs

Circuit Training: This is a total body program that generally uses light resistances (e.g. 12-20 RM or 40% to 60% 1 RM). The person moves from exercise to exercise with little rest. Generally 9-15 exercises make up a circuit but this can vary. This program ensures that no muscle group receives too much stress and is appropriate for beginners and for many medical issues. Machines, free weights or a combination can make up the circuit as can exercise tubing, stability balls etc. Circuit training will improve not only aerobic capacity but strength and some power as well.

Split Routine Programs: Split routines split training into separate days. Each day, a different body part is worked. For example, one might have a "chest and back day". The downside is that these routines may require more days working out. This may not be the best program for novices. One study looked at 5 months of training with either a total body program or a split routine in 30 untrained young women.[29] Both programs, showed similar strength gains.

Super Set Programs: A superset, can refer to two different types of programs. One type of involves performing two exercises back to back that targets opposing muscle groups. For example, one might perform a leg extension followed by a leg curl. Little/no rest is taken between exercises. Another type involves performing 2 or 3 different exercises for the same muscle group with little rest. For example, one might do a set of biceps curls, followed by a set of preacher curls.

Interval Training Programs: This program, sometimes called "HIT" (High Intensity Training) is often used with aerobic exercise but it can be applied to strength training as well. Here, people alternate between intense and less intense efforts. For example, one might bike ride at a high level for 30 seconds, followed by a lower level for 2 minutes. In theory, interval training may decrease injuries by reducing the overall time muscles are subjected to high degrees of stress. Interval training can also improve aerobic fitness levels. This program might also result in more calories being used in a workout. As a general rule, make the rest period 2 to 3 times as long as the work period. So, if the person runs on a treadmill for 1 minute, that person should walk for 2 to 3 minutes. Because it's intense, it's not appropriate for beginners or those with a variety of health issues.

Pyramiding Programs: In this program, the lifter usually begins with a light resistance that he/she can lift for about 10-12 reps. The lifter then increases the weight (by 2.5-10 lbs). This continues until the lifter can only perform one rep (the top of the pyramid). Then, the weight is reduced (by 2.5-10 lbs), resulting in more reps being able to be performed. At the bottom of the pyramid, the lifter is once again, back to his/her starting point. In a variation, the lifter performs only half the pyramid. This is where we get terms like "up pyramiding" and "down pyramiding". Which way is better? Little research proves one way is better than another. For beginners, performing either program will be difficult, resulting in DOMS and, in theory, may ramp up injuries.

Negatives: In this program, the lifter only does eccentric muscle actions (negatives). Performing only eccentric reps is an advanced program and may result in injury (muscle tearing away from the bone) if used in beginners. This program is not appropriate for those with a variety of health issues.

Super Slow Programs: Here, the weight is lifted very slowly. For example, it might take 10 seconds to lift the weight and 10 seconds to lower the weight. Some research suggests that this program may improve strength in beginners.[32] Other research hints that super slow may not be the best for weight loss in experienced lifter's because fewer calories may be used.[31.] On the other hand, in theory, super slow programs may lead to fewer injuries.

Common Fitness Tests

The following are overviews of common tests that trainers can use to measure various fitness components. These are not the only tests available. Fitness software programs also exist which can help trainers record, analyze and track progress made.

Muscular Strength

10RM Test. After proper warm up determine the most weight that can be lifted on the bench press (and/or leg press) only 10 times with good form.

Muscle Endurance

Timed Pushups. After proper warm up, the person performs as many pushups with good form as possible within 1 minute. Resting is allowed but the clock does not stop during rest periods. The test may be contraindicated in those with injuries to low back or shoulders and those who cannot perform a push up.

Times Sit ups. Perform as many sit ups (or crunches) as possible in 1 minute. Resting is allowed but the clock does not stop during rest periods. Contraindicated in persons with osteoporosis as well as those with low back and neck injuries and those not strong enough to get up from floor.

Cardiovascular Endurance

3 Minute Step Test. Person steps up & down at a specific rate for 3 minutes. The pulse is taken before/after the test and entered into an equation which yields the result.

Rockport Walking Test. Person walks 1 mile as fast as possible. The pulse is taken immediately after the test and is entered into an equation which gives the result.

Treadmill Fitness Test. Some computerized treadmills have a "Fitness Test". The treadmill measures pulse and provides a score.

Flexibility

Sit and Reach Test. Following a warm up, the person sits on the floor with legs straight and reaches forward, bending at the hips. The trainer measures how far they can reach forward. The best of 3 trials is recorded. Bouncing is not allowed.

Body Composition Tests

Bioelectric Impedance Analysis (BIA). Most gyms have a portable BIA device. The person holds the device with arms in front. A small electrical signal is passed through the body. Because fat is a poor conductor of electricity, the slower the current travels, the higher the percent body fat. The test accuracy depends on many factors including not eating/drinking or exercising for at least 12 hrs prior to the test and refraining from alcohol for at least 48 hrs. For safety, this test should not be used in those who have pacemakers/defibrillators or in pregnant women.

Skin Fold Testing. Special calipers are used to *pinch* the person at various sites on their body. Testing only occurs on the right side of the body. The averages of the sites are used to estimate body fat. While accurate if performed correctly, most health clubs do not use this method.

Underwater Weighing. The person is dunked completely under water and weighed. This, along with their weight on the land is used to calculate body composition. Often called the "gold standard" because it's very accurate, most health clubs do not have the equipment to perform this test.

Bod Pod. The person sits in a special chamber which measures air displacement. The technician can determine body composition in minutes. The accuracy is very close to underwater weighing. The Bod Pod is very expensive so most health clubs may not have it.

Basic Health Tests

In addition to fitness testing, personal trainers may also perform various other tests which can help identify disease risk. This information can help the trainer design a better program by allowing not only attainment of current goals but also by possibly helping the client avoid illness/disease in the future.

Resting Heart Rate (RHR). Measurement of RHR in some cases can help the trainer identify if a client has been exercising regularly and in athletes, identify over training syndrome. An average RHR can vary from 60 bpm - 100 bpm. Note, persons on medications for CAD and/or HTN may appear to have a lower than average RHR but this is due to the medications they take.

Blood Pressure. The measurement of blood pressure (BP) should be performed on all new clients who have high blood pressure, ideally before and after exercise so the trainer can see how exercise is effecting their condition. Measurement of blood pressure as a general test may also draw attention to high blood pressure in those who are unaware of it.

Body Mass Index (BMI). If you know the bodyweight and how tall a person is you can calculate Body Mass Index. BMI is useful as a quick test of a person's disease risk because many obesity-related problems increase as BMI increases over 25 kg/m^2. One common equation used to calculate BMI is :   BMI = 703 (weight in pounds ÷ height^2 in inches).

BMI	Meaning
18.5-24.9	Healthy weight
25-29.9	Overweight
> 30	Obese

Abdominal Circumference. Those who carry most of their weight around the belly are at elevated risk of obesity related conditions. Research finds that men who have a waist circumference greater than 40 inches (102 cm) and women whose waist is greater than 35 inches (88 cm) are at higher risk of heart disease, type II diabetes, hypertension, high cholesterol and other obesity related issues.[33] Measurement is at the narrowest part of the waist, usually a little bit above the belly button, after a normal exhalation. Sometimes people appear to be "normal" according to BMI yet have a high waist circumference measurement. Thus, this can be a very useful test to do.

CHAPTER 6
Determining Exercise Intensity

Fitness trainers must be able to determine how hard people are exercising so they can design safe programs and modify them as needed. Fortunately there are many ways to do this. Fitness trainers should be familiar with these different methods because only knowing one or two ways may not suit all of their clients.

Using Heart Rate To Determine Exercise Intensity

The most common method. Basically the maximum heart rate is calculated and from this the trainer calculates a "target heart rate" which they feel is safe and appropriate for the client. The maximum heart rate (MHR) is determined from this equation: 220 - Age. So, if a person was 50 years old, their maximum heart rate would be 220 - 50 = 170 beats per minute (bpm). Once this is known, the trainer selects two percentages of this number, a higher and lower percentage. Those are multiplied by maximum heart rate to determine the target heart rate range (THR). For example, suppose you wanted the person in the example to exercise between 60% and 80% of their maximum heart rate. In this example it would be:

$$170\text{bpm} \times 0.6 = \textbf{102 bpm} \qquad \& \qquad 170 \times 0.8 = \textbf{136 bpm}$$

So in this example, you would have the person maintain a heart rate of between 102 and 136 bpm when they were exercising aerobically. But, how do you determine what percentages are best for the person? Essentially you are going to make an educated guess. This will be based on the person's current fitness level, health of the person and any medical conditions they have. Generally most experts recommend that healthy people exercise at an intensity of between 60% and 80% to 85% of maximum heart rate, but for people with health problems (e.g. arthritis) the guideline can be lower. This is why using 60% - 85% won't always work. Another thing to remember is that the 220 - Age equation only estimates maximum heart rate. The "real" maximum heart rate might be 10-12 beats above or below what 220 - Age determines. One major problem with this method is that it will not be accurate in persons who take medications for high blood pressure.

Karvonen Heart Rate Method

This is often said to be a more accurate than the method just described. Here, we must first know the persons resting heart rate (RHR) and their age. To get a the RHR, have the person rest quietly for 5-10 minutes. They should have no caffeine or tobacco for at least 30 minutes before you take their pulse. Take their pulse at the radial side of the wrist for a full minute. The Karvonen formula has 4 steps:

Karvonen Heart Rate Steps

Step 1:   Subtract age from 220

Step 2:   Subtract RHR from step 1

Step 3:   Multiply the result of step 2 by two percentages

Step 4:   Add RHR to the results of step 3

Karvonen Formula Example: Your client is a 50 year old man with a RHR of 45 bpm. Based on their health history, you estimate that they should exercise aerobically at an intensity of 70% - 85%.

Step 1. $220 - 50 = 170$ bpm

Step 2. 170 bpm $- 45$ bpm $= 125$ bpm

Step 3. $125 \times .07 = 87$ & $125 \times 0.85 = 106$

Step 4. $87 + 45 =$ **132 bpm**   & $106 = 45 =$ **151 bpm**

Answer. You instruct the person to maintain 132 to 151 bpm when they are doing cardio.

In general, a RHR can range from 60 bpm to 100 bpm. Regular aerobic exercise tends to lower RHR. In the example above, one might assume that a RHR of 45 bpm was the result of regular workouts. However it might also be the result of medications taken to treat heart disease or high blood pressure. These conditions are abbreviated CAD and HTN respectively. These medications (e.g. beta blockers) artificially slow RHR to help regulate the medical condition. Trainers should not use heart rate to determine exercise intensity in people taking these medications. Doing so will lead to not only inaccuracies but medical emergencies as well. Options to use with these individuals include the RPE scale and the Talk Test.

RPE Scale

RPE stands for Ratings of Perceived Exertion. Here, the person rates their exertion level on a scale from zero to 10. A rating of zero means "nothing at all" and a rating of "10" represents a full out, maximal effort. Another name for the RPE Scale is the Borg Scale. One advantage of the RPE scale is that it can be used for both aerobic exercise and anaerobic exercise. For example, you might ask someone how heavy a weight feels on a scale from zero to 10. The RPE scale works well for people with high blood pressure, novices and children.

RPE Scale

Rating	Meaning
0	Nothing at all
1	Very weak effort
2	Weak effort
3	Moderately strong or difficult effort
5	Strong or difficult effort
7	Very strong or difficult effort
10	Maximum effort

Talk Test

The talk test is based on the premise that a person should be able to talk when working out aerobically. If they can't talk they are exercising too hard. This method works well with beginners, children, those with medical issues and people who don't understand how to use the RPE Scale.

VO2max

VO2 stands for the "volume of oxygen". More precisely, it's the volume of oxygen we use to make energy (ATP) aerobically. So it's really a measure of how good our aerobic energy system is working! VO2max is the maximum volume of oxygen that we can use to make energy aerobically. When we are exercising at VO2max, our aerobic energy system is working at its maximum capacity. When we exercise at an intensity above VO2max, the anaerobic energy system starts to contribute more to our energy needs. This can result in the buildup of metabolites (e.g. lactate) which can reduce our exercise performance. Aerobic capacity begins to decrease significantly after the age of 45. This can increase the risk for heart disease and other disorders. Factors that can reduce VO2max include age, cardiovascular health, genetics and poor lifestyle behaviors. Aerobic exercise can help slow this decline and even improve aerobic capacity in many people. Trainers usually don't measure VO2 but they may estimate percentages of VO2max with METs and the Karvonen formula.

Metabolic Equivalents (METs)

Metabolism can be defined as the speed we burn calories. METs allows us compare our metabolic rate during exercise to what it is when we are sleeping. Sleeping is our lowest metabolic rate (BMR) and is defined as 1 MET. So, if you are on a treadmill and it says you are at 12 METs, it means your metabolism is 12 times higher than when sleeping. It also means that you're' burning calories 12 times faster than when sleeping.

An intensity of 1 MET is equal to 3.5 milliliters of oxygen per kilogram of bodyweight per minute. A kilogram is equal to 2.2 pounds. Both METs and VO2 are really the same. METs is just an easier way of expressing VO2. Because we know the value of 1 MET, it's possible to estimate VO2 for a given exercise intensity. For example, if you were on a treadmill and the readout said you were at 10 METs, that means your VO2 at that moment is 10 x 3.5 = 35 ml O2/kg BW/min.

METs can be a valuable tool but remember the client's initial fitness level and health issues really determine what MET level is best and safest. Use RPE sale and the Talk Test also to get a better picture of how hard they are exercising. Never rely on one method only.

CHAPTER 7

Weightlifting Exercises

We will now review how to properly perform and spot a variety of strength training exercises. This chapter will also review the major muscles used for each exercise as well as "tricks of the trade", to take you *beyond the basics* so you can outperform other trainers.

Barbell Bench Press

Primary Muscles Worked: Pectoralis major and minor, anterior deltoids, triceps, serratus anterior.

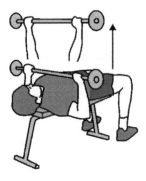

> **Quick Tip:** Retract the shoulder blades prior to doing this exercise with heavy weights.

Exercise Technique: The barbell should be secured by collars. There should be a slight bend in the elbows when you grasp the barbell while on the bench and the barbell should be lined up with the eyes. The body should be evenly distributed on the bench with feet on floor at least shoulder width apart. Grasp barbell with a pronated grip, wrapping the thumbs around the bar. The grip should be about shoulder-width apart or a little wider. The wrists are straight and not bent. Hands and elbows are in line with each other. Begin by lifting the barbell off of its suspension hooks to a position in line with the chest. Arms are straight but elbows are not locked. Eccentric phase: Lower the bar slowly, stopping when the elbow is at the level of the shoulder. At the end of the eccentric phase the forearms should be perpendicular to the ground (i.e., 90° bend in arms). Do not bounce the barbell off of the chest. Pause for a second. Concentric phase: Slowly press the barbell upward and stop just before the elbows are locked out. Repeat for the desired number of repetitions.

Spotting: The trainer is behind the head of the lifter during this exercise. The trainer should be in the athletic position (abs tight, knees slightly bent). Trainers should ask if the lifter needs a "lift off" or help getting the barbell off the hooks to its proper location over the chest. If yes, spotters often use an *alternated grip* (one hand is supinated; the other pronated). The same grip is used to help re-rack the barbell at the end of the set. At some point during the concentric phase the lifter may reach the *sticking point* (the most difficult point of the exercise). The lifter may need help during this time.

Spotters should always ask the lifter how many reps he/she can perform so they have an idea when the lifter may need help. Remove weight plates from the barbell evenly. Taking too much weight off only one side may cause the barbell to flip over and cause serious injury.

Comments & Suggestions: The technique described above is commonly performed by many people; but, in some cases, this may result in rotator cuff shoulder injury. Thus, a more narrow grip is sometimes advocated.[34] An added bonus to a narrow grip is that it also tends to place more emphasis on the pecs than does a wider grip. The barbell does not need to touch the chest. Doing so may cause or exacerbate shoulder injuries. When calculating weight lifted, remember to count the Olympic bar and collars.

Common Bench Press Mistakes

Error	Explanation
Lifting too much weight	Golgi tendon organ (GTO) relaxes muscles if lifting too much weight
Bouncing barbell off chest	Barbell might crack sternum or cause other injury. The lifter did not properly perform the eccentric phase of the exercise.
Lifting too fast	Places excessive stress on joints, increasing injury risk
Not wrapping thumbs around bar	Barbell might roll out of hands
Arching the low back	Places excessive stress on low back muscles and spinal cord
Bending wrists	Places excessive forces on delicate wrist bones
Raising head off of bench	Stresses cervical neck area. May cause neck injury
Shoulders arching to earlobes (seated chest press)	Incorrect technique. May signify shoulders performing more work than they should.
Holding breath	Valsalva Maneuver. Might increases BP to dangerous levels
Grip too wide	The wider the grip the more stress on the shoulders
Locking out elbows	May increase injury to elbow joint

Dumbbell Bench Press

Primary Muscles Used: Pectoralis major and minor, anterior deltoids, triceps, serratus anterior.

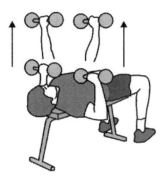

> **Quick Tip:** During the eccentric phase, stop when the elbows are at or just a little below the shoulders.

Exercise Technique: Grasp two equal weighted dumbbells and sit on a stable exercise bench with dumbbells resting on your thighs. If needed, perform hip flexion of the thighs to help lift the dumbbells to shoulder level prior to lying supine on the bench. Lie supine on the bench, with feet on floor at least shoulder width apart, if not wider. Head, shoulders and buttocks should be evenly distributed on the bench. Wrists should be straight, not bent. The dumbbells should be at chest level, aligned with the nipple line. Keep the thumbs wrapped around the dumbbells. That elbows are pointed away from the body. The elbows should be at the level of the shoulders. The forearms should be perpendicular to floor. <u>Concentric phase</u>: Slowly press dumbbells upward. Don't allow the dumbbells to sway back or forth or lose control of them at any point in the ROM. Press until soft lockout is reached. Do not arch the low back or remove the feet from the floor during the lift. <u>Eccentric phase</u>: Slowly lower the dumbbells to the starting point and repeat for the desired number of repetitions. At the end of the exercise at the bottom of the last eccentric phase, rotate the elbows inward toward the body, sit up slowly and rest the dumbbells on the thighs.

Spotting: Trainers should be positioned behind the lifters head. Ask the lifter how he/she wants to be spotted ahead of time. During the eccentric phase trainers may place their hands at the height of the shoulders to cue the lifter not to lower his/her elbows past this point. During the concentric phase, trainers may grasp the wrists of the client to help him/her steady the dumbbells and reduce injury. Do not pull the dumbbells up by the wrists of the lifter. This can result in shoulder injury especially if the lifter is not expecting it. With very heavy dumbbells it may be necessary to hand the lifter the dumbbells prior to performing the exercise. If this occurs, the spotter should *not* hold the dumbbell by the handgrip. This prevents the lifter from grasping the dumbbell safely. Instead, grasp each end of the dumbbell and hand it to the lifter.

Comments & Suggestions: The lifter should maintain a closed-grip on dumbbells at all times during the exercise. This will reduce injury. A bench that is too high may cause the lifter to arch the lower back. If this happens, place the feet on a raised platform to alleviate this problem. Placing the feet on the bench is an option but in this position, the lifter's base of support is narrower which might lead to falling off the bench. Lifter's sometimes lower the dumbbells to points where the elbows are below the torso. They do this because they want to "feel the stretch." But, this practice removes stress from the chest muscles and places more stress on the shoulder joint. This can increase shoulder injuries. This exercise can also be performed with a neutral grip where the elbows are closer to the body and palms facing each other. This grip generally places less stress on the shoulder. Do not drop the weights on the floor while supine on the bench. This can lead to shoulder injury. Technically, dumbbells are more difficult to lift than barbells.

Pushups On The Stability Ball

Primary Muscles Used: Pectoralis major, anterior deltoids, triceps, serratus anterior, posterior deltoids, rectus abdominis, core musculature.

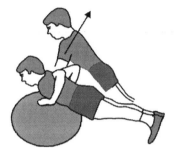

> **Quick Tip:** Be able to do regular push-ups first. Feet closer together increases the difficulty.

Exercise Technique: Place the hands on the top outer, upper sides of the stability ball, about shoulder width apart with fingers oriented downward. The legs are extended and at shoulder width apart or wider with bodyweight on toes. Eccentric phase: Slowly lower the upper torso toward the ball while keeping the ball in line with the chest. Halt the movement when the elbows are at the level of the torso or when comfortable. Concentric phase: Press down on the ball, lifting the torso to starting point, while again, keeping the ball in line with the chest. Stop just before the elbows lock out. Hold position for a second or two. Repeat.

Spotting: The low back should not slouch downward. The head should stay neutral, neither lifting up nor turning to the sides. The hands may slide off the ball if sweaty.

Comments & Suggestions: This is an advanced form of pushups that challenges the entire core musculature and requires considerable strength and endurance. This can also be an effective shoulder stabilizing exercise for overall shoulder health. Novices often believe the core is just the abs however, the it really includes all the muscles of the trunk. Another version of this exercise is to perform the push up with hands on the floor and ankles or toes on the ball. One limiting factor to performing this movement may be on the forces experienced on the wrists.

Pec Deck (Machine Pec Fly

Primary Muscles Used: Pectoralis major, anterior deltoid

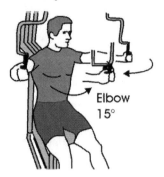

Elbow
15°

> **Quick Tip:** Some versions double as a reverse fly machine. Make sure the handles are properly oriented before using.

Exercise Technique: Adjust the movable arms of the machine and seat so that the handles are aligned with the nipple line of the chest. Sit facing away from the machine and grasp the handles with a closed grip. The elbows should be slightly bent. Wrists should be ridged and not hyper-flexed. Concentric phase: Slowly bring the handles together in a controlled fashion, stopping just before the hands touch. Eccentric phase: Slowly release to starting position and repeat.

Spotting: Trainers should ensure that the seat is at the proper height and that the elbows are slightly bent. Elbows do not go behind the torso during the eccentric phase of the exercise.

Comments & Suggestions. Remind people that many machines can double as a rear delt machine by altering the range of motion pins which are usually located near the top of the device. People often don't know this and so they reach too far back. This can lead to shoulder injuries. Tell people also that greater ROM does not always mean greater chest development. Avoid this exercise in people with shoulder injuries.

Prone Reverse Fly With Stabilty Ball

Primary Muscles Used: Posterior deltoids, latissimus dorsi, rhomboids, rotator cuff.

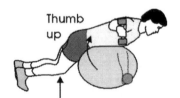

Thumb
up

> **Quick Tip:** Use a bench if a stability ball is not available.

Exercise Technique: Obtain two light and equal weighted dumbbells and lay prone on a stability ball with the ball at the naval. The legs are extended about hip to shoulder width apart with a slight bend at the knees. The head is neutral and the abs contracted. The exercise starts with the arms extended outward from the body (maintain a slight bend at the elbows) below the plane of the torso. The hands are oriented such that the thumbs are pointed up. Concentric phase: Slowly, raise the arms upward while keeping the shoulder blades pulled together. Stop when the arms are about shoulder height. Eccentric phase: Slowly return arms to starting position. Repeat.

Spotting: The head stays neutral. The shoulder blades remain contracted. The trunk does not round forward over the ball. In beginners, you may need to hold the ankles for added stability.

Comments & Suggestions: This is a good rear deltoid exercise and can help strengthen the rotator cuff. This exercise can also be performed without dumbbells. In this instance, the thumbs should point up to the ceiling. An easier, albeit equally effective, version of this exercise is performed with knees bent and on the floor.

Seated Row Machine

Primary Muscles Used: Latissimus dorsi, rhomboids, trapezius, posterior deltoids.

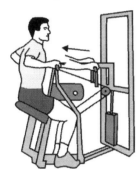

> **Quick Tip:** Pull the shoulder blades together before pulling the weight back.

Exercise Technique: Adjust the seat of the machine so that the chest is against the chest pad when seated and the arms are about parallel with the floor. If the machine has an adjustable chest pad, adjust it so that the lifter can reach the handles comfortably yet still have a slight bend in the elbows. Concentric phase: Grasp handles with neutral grip. Retract shoulder blades and pull backward until elbows are under shoulders. Hold for a second. Eccentric phase: Slowly return to the starting position while maintaining shoulder blade retraction. Repeat.

Spotting: Stand behind the lifter and place your finger between his/her shoulder blades to prompt them into retraction. Have him/her imagine what they would do if you dropped an ice cube down their back. If the shoulders roll forward, it's a sign the weight may be too heavy or the lifter is not holding shoulder blades together. The lifter should not rock back and forth during the movement.

Comments & Suggestions: Trainers often advise lifter's to retract their shoulders blades and hold the retraction throughout the movement. But is this always best? For heavier loads, yes, because it allows better trunk and shoulder stabilization. For lighter loads, though, (e.g., 15 or more reps) holding the retraction may not be as important. In this situation, retracting and releasing the shoulder blades after each rep offers variety to the exercise. Rocking back and forth is not necessary and may strain the low back. Rather, maintain the torso in an upright posture throughout the exercise. The neutral grip is usually preferable to a pronated grip for those with shoulder injuries.

Lat Pull Down

Primary Muscles Used: Latissimus dorsi, posterior deltoid, rhomboids, teres major, trapezius.

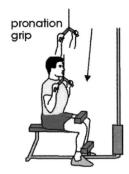

pronation grip

> **Quick Tip:** Pull the shoulder blades together prior to pulling the bar downward.

Exercise Technique: Sit facing the lat pull down machine and grasp the bar with over handed grip (pronated grip). Hand placement on the bar can vary according to individual biomechanics and current/previous injuries, but in general the hands are at shoulder width apart or a little wider. There should be a slight bend in the elbows and the elbows are pointed outward. Lean back slightly and retract shoulder blades. Concentric phase: Slowly pull the bar downward to the front of the head. Stop when the upper arms are about parallel with the floor. Hold for a second. Eccentric phase: Slowly let the bar rise to the starting position and repeat. Do not let the bar go so high that the elbows lock out. Maintain slight bend in elbows. Repeat for the desired number of reps.

Spotting: The spotter stands behind the lifter and makes sure that the lifter is performing the exercise correctly. During heavy lifts, always retract shoulder blades. With lighter lifts, holding the retraction may not be needed. Slightly leaning back is ok but excessive lean or rocking back and forth is not.

Comments & Suggestions: Pulling the bar behind the head is controversial because it may increase the risk of shoulder injury.[36] It is generally felt by physical therapists and orthopedic surgeons that pulling to the front is safer. People sometimes use a very wide grip to target the "outer lats." However, there is no such thing as *outer or inner lats*. This practice may increase shoulder injury risk. A variation of this exercise is to only retract the shoulder blades without pulling with the arms.

Dumbbell One Arm Bent Over Row

Primary Muscles Used: Posterior deltoids, latissimus dorsi, rhomboids, teres major.

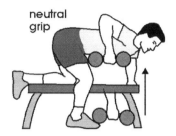

neutral grip

> **Quick Tip:** Retract the shoulder blade prior to pulling with the arm. The head should be neutral.

Exercise Technique: Obtain a dumbbell and place one knee on the exercise bench (the lower leg will also rest on the bench). The other foot is on the floor, pointed straight ahead with knee slightly bent. The hand that will not grasp the dumbbell is placed on the front or side of the exercise bench for stability. The trunk will be about parallel with the bench. The body weight should be evenly distributed between the bent knee and hand. The head should be neutral, neither looking up or to the sides. Grasp the dumbbell with a neutral grip. Abs should be contracted slightly. <u>Concentric phase</u>: With the dumbbell in line with the shoulders, retract the shoulder blade and slowly pull the dumbbell upward until a 90° bend at the elbow is reached (at this point the upper arm is parallel with the floor). <u>Eccentric phase</u>: Slowly lower the dumbbell to the starting position while maintaining retraction of the shoulder blade. Do not lock out the elbow at the bottom of the eccentric phase. The dumbbell should stay close to the body at all times. Repeat for the desired number of reps.

Spotting: People often twist the trunk in the direction of the pull in an attempt to help them lift the weight. This is cheating due to lifting too much weight. Rather, the chest should be facing down toward the floor. The head should stay neutral, neither looking upward or to the sides.

Comments & Suggestions: While a flat bench is shown here, an adjustable bench elevated to about 30° can also be used. The knee and hand used for support should both be from the same side of the body. That is, if the left knee is bent, stabilize with the left hand and vice versa. People with high blood pressure or heart disease may get dizzy after rising up from this exercise. This exercise may aggravate existing low back problems.

Machine Shoulder Press

Primary Muscles Used: Anterior and medial deltoids, triceps, trapezius.

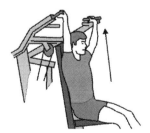

> **Quick Tip**: Grasping the handles with palms facing each other reduces the stress on the shoulders and possible injury.

Exercise Technique: The seat should be adjusted so that the thighs are about parallel with the floor. In the starting position, the bent elbows should be about shoulder height or a little lower. The trainer may need to lower the seat height. The shoulders are weaker when the elbows are lower than shoulder height. This reduces the amount of weight that can be lifted. When the handles are grasped with a closed, pronated grip, the elbows should be pointing out from the sides of the body. The wrists are not bent. <u>Concentric phase</u>: Press upward until soft lockout is reached. <u>Eccentric phase</u>: Slowly lower until elbows are at shoulder height. Repeat for the desired number of repetitions.

Spotting: Common errors during this exercise include excessive arching of the low back; hands too far apart; turning the head during the lift and not keeping feet on the floor. People often hold their breath (Valsalva maneuver) which is not recommended.

Comments & Suggestions: Use caution with this exercise if the lifter has any neck, shoulder or elbow injuries. If performed with a barbell, pressing the bar behind the head may result in rotator cuff injuries. Many shoulder press machines allow this exercise to be performed with a neutral grip (i.e., palms of hands facing each other), which is usually considered safer for the shoulders. Keep loads light if the person has high blood pressure and ensure they do not do Valsalva. Use with caution in those with rotator cuff issues.

The Rotator Cuff

The rotator cuff represents four muscles that keep the upper arm bone (humerus) in its socket and is very active during all shoulder exercises. The muscles of the rotator cuff are the supraspinatus, infraspinatus, subscapularis and teres minor. Rotator cuff injuries are common in baseball, tennis, basketball, weightlifting, swimming or any activity where the arms are regularly raised over the head.

Common signs include shoulder pain especially when reaching over the head or when lifting weights (e.g., bench pressing, push-ups or shoulder press) or when reaching the arm behind the back. Sometimes the pain occurs when not moving and may even cause almost total lack of movement in the arm. In extreme cases there may be a tear of the rotator cuff which may require surgery. Usual treatment includes ice to relive inflammation, resting the area and halting the activity which caused the injury. A physician may inject steroids (e.g., cortisone) into the area, prescribe pain relievers and refer the person to a physical therapist who can recommend various exercises (e.g., external shoulder rotation) to help strengthen the rotator cuff.

External Shoulder Rotation With Dumbbell

Primary Muscles Used: Rotator Cuff Muscles (primarily infraspinatus and teres minor).

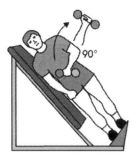

> **Quick Tip:** For added difficulty, perform on the floor.

Exercise Technique: Obtain a light dumbbell and lie on your side, on a stable incline exercise board (or floor or flat bench for added difficulty). The arm to be used should be bent at 90°. <u>Concentric phase</u>: Rotate the bent arm outward from the body, stopping close to the end of pain-free normal ROM . <u>Eccentric phase</u>: Slowly lower to the starting position and repeat.

Spotting: A common error is moving the elbow away from the body. Having the lifter hold a towel between the elbow and torso should eliminate this from occurring as well as increase the blood supply to the muscle. Alternately, the spotter may place one or two fingers on the elbow to remind the lifter of the proper position.

Comments & Suggestions: People are usually stronger doing *internal shoulder rotation* than external rotation. As such, an imbalance between these muscles might contribute to shoulder instability. There are several variations of this exercise. The version shown in the picture is less intense than that usually performed (on the floor). The exercise can also be performed standing, using elastic tubing. For very bad pain start with isometrics against a wall. Normally, external and internal rotations are performed with lighter resistances and higher number of reps (e.g., 15-20 reps).

Shoulder Flexion With Dumbbells

Primary Muscles Used: Anterior deltoid, pectoralis major.

Neutral
grip

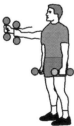

> **Quick Tip:** Performing with exercise tubing or a cable machine may strengthen the muscles over a greater ROM than dumbbells.

Exercise Technique: Obtain two equal weighted dumbbells and stand with feet shoulder width apart with a slight bend in the knees and hips. The dumbbells should be at sides, held with neutral grip. There should be a slight bend in the elbows at all times. Concentric phase: Slowly raise dumbbells up and in front of the body while maintaining a slight bend at the elbows. Stop when hands are at about shoulder level (i.e., parallel with floor). Eccentric phase: Slowly lower to starting position. Repeat for desired number of reps.

Spotting: The lifter should look straight ahead. The dumbbells should not tilt down at the wrists. If this wrists bend it may mean that the weight is too heavy for the lifter.

Comments & Suggestions: This exercise is also known as the front raise. Some lifter's perform this exercise with a pronated (palms down) grip, which reduces the influence of the biceps muscles. Because the shoulder is relatively easy to injure and because this is a single joint exercise, keep the weight light. This exercise can also be performed seated or with exercise tubing or a cable machine.

Barbell Shrug

Primary Muscles Used: Upper trapezius, rhomboids, levator scapulae.

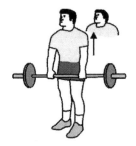

> **Quick Tip:** Remember to keep a slight bend at the knees during this exercise.

Exercise Technique: Hold an equal weighted barbell in front of the body (it can be behind the body as well). Hands are pronated and at shoulder width or a little wider. Elbows are slightly bent. There should be a slight bend in the knees. The lifter will now have a slight forward lean which is ok. Concentric phase: Slowly raise the shoulders upward. In this position, the shoulders will travel slightly behind the neck. This is ok. Eccentric phase: Slowly lower the barbell to the starting point while maintaining a slight bend at the elbows. Repeat for desired number of repetitions.

Spotting: The lifter's head should look straight ahead and not turn. There should be a small bend in the knees and the lifter should be slightly leaning forward which helps to better recruit the muscles used.

Comments & Suggestions: This exercise can also be performed with dumbbells. It is not necessary to roll the shoulders while performing this exercise. Doing so is usually not needed because it does not effectively work the muscles optimally.

Controversial Exercises: Use With Caution

Upright rows	May increase risk of shoulder injuries
Behind head military press	May increase risk of shoulder injuries
Behind head lat pull down	May increase risk of shoulder injuries
Good Mornings	May increase risk of low back injuries
Deep knee squats (>90°)	May increase risk of knee injuries

Supine Leg Press Machine

Primary Muscles Used: Quadriceps (vastus lateralis, vastus medialis, vastus intermedius, rectus femoris), hamstrings (semimembranosus, semitendinosus,, biceps femoris), gluteal muscles.

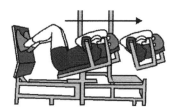

> **Quick Tip:** Keeping the toes at least as high as knees works more of the hamstrings and butt muscles.

Exercise Technique: Adjust the machine to the appropriate weight and recline with shoulders under the pads and feet on the metal platform. Feet should be at hip width apart with toes pointed up or slightly outward. Toes are at least as high as knees if not a little higher. Concentric phase: Press feet into the foot plate, lifting the weight stack and halting just before full knee lock out occurs (i.e., perform a soft lock out). Eccentric phase: Slowly lower the weight stack, halting just before the weights touch. Repeat for the desired number of reps.

Spotting: Ensure that the lifter's feet are at least as high as his/her knees and that the back is not arching. The spotter also reminds the lifter to breathe during the activity.

Comments & Suggestions: The supine leg press is one of several types of this exercise. All variations basically challenge the same muscle groups. A common mistake is performing the exercise with the knees placed higher than the toes. This puts perpendicular forces (sheering forces) on the knees and can increase pain/injury. Another common mistake is letting the knees bow inward during the lift. The knees should be at about hip or shoulder width apart during the lift. Arching the low back may occur on the supine leg press when the lifter attempts to lift more weight than he/she can handle. If this occurs, reduce the resistance and lift that load slower or alternatively, move to another type of leg press.

Squat (With stability ball)

Primary Muscles Used: Quadriceps (vastus lateralis, vastus medialis, vastus intermedius, rectus femoris), hamstrings (semimembranosus, semitendinosus,, biceps femoris), gluteal muscles, calves.

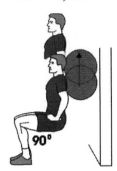

Quick Tip: For added difficulty, use dumbbells and/or combine with biceps curl, lateral raise or shoulder press.

Exercise Technique: The stability ball should be placed at about the lower back region. Feet should be about shoulder width apart with toes pointing straight ahead. There should be a slight bend in the knees. Eccentric phase: Slowly lower the body (as if sitting down in a chair), being mindful not to increase the forward lean of the torso during the descent nor to let the knees travel past the toes. Descend to approximately 60° to 90° or to where comfortable. Concentric phase: Slowly rise up to starting position, halting the movement just before the knees lock out. Repeat for the desired number of reps.

Spotting: Ensure that the knees don't travel in front of the toes when viewed from the side. If the this happens, bring the feet further out from the wall and/or instruct the person to "push your butt into the wall." The knees should not bow inward.

Comments & Suggestions: Make sure the person can do a wall squat and /or has sufficient balance before introducing the stability ball. For added difficulty, dumbbells, elastic tubing, or other forms of resistance may be used. Advising people to "press through the heels" places greater emphasis on the glutes. Squats are a functional exercise but they may aggravate osteoarthritis pain in some people.

Squat With Barbell

Primary Muscles Used: Quadriceps (vastus lateralis, vastus medialis, vastus intermedius, rectus femoris), hamstrings (semimembranosus, semitendinosus, biceps femoris), gluteal muscles.

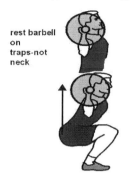

rest barbell on traps-not neck

Quick Tip: Don't let knees go past toes. Look straight ahead— not upward to the ceiling.

Exercise Technique: Load an equally weighted barbell onto a power rack that has been adjusted to be at shoulder height or a little lower (this will allow the lifter to pick up and re-rack the weight easier). Stand under the bar with feet about shoulder or hip width apart and pointed straight ahead. The bar should rest on the upper back and posterior deltoids near the trapezius and be grasped a little wider than shoulder width with a closed pronated grip. In this position, the elbows are pointed outward from and behind the body to help keep the weight on the upper back. The weight should be evenly distributed over this area. Pull shoulder blades together. The head looks straight ahead (not up to the ceiling). Now, lift the weight upward by extending at the hips and knees. The barbell is now resting freely on the upper body. Take a step or two backward in preparation for the eccentric phase of the lift. Feet are still about shoulder to hip width apart and pointed straight ahead. Eccentric phase: Flex at the hips and knees and slowly lower the body, remembering not to lean too far forward. Stop the decent when about 60°-90° of knee flexion is reached (at 90° the thighs will be about parallel with the floor). Hold for a second. Concentric phase: Extend at the hips and knees (as getting up from a chair) to a standing position, being conscious not to lock out the knees at the top of the movement. Repeat for the desired number of reps.

Spotting: Ensure the knees do not go past the toes and that the lifter does not descend lower than 90° or where he/she feels comfortable. If the heels come off the floor, the lifter has gone too low for their level of flexibility. The knees should remain the same distance apart during the lift and should not bow inward or outward. Technically, at least two people should spot the squat —one on each end of the bar. This way, each spotter can cup their hands together and grasp the end of the barbell to easily help with lift-offs or if the lifter needs assistance.

Comments & Suggestions: The technique described here is different than for powerlifting and other competitive weightlifting events where squatting lower than 90° may be necessary. Lower body flexibility impacts the ability to perform the squat. Inflexibility in the lower body can contribute to the compression forces on the spine. Placing blocks or weight plates under the heels can increase the stress on the knees. Performing barbell squats with those who have osteoporosis may lead to crushing of the spinal cord bones.

Squatting: Top 18 Mistakes to Avoid

Common Mistake	Explanation
Placing blocks/plates under heels	Increases stress on knees
Squatting below 90 degrees	In theory, this may increase injury to knees
Resting barbell on cervical spine	Weight might fracture cervical spinal bones
Bouncing at bottom of exercise	Increases stress on knee joints and low back
Performing reps too fast	Increases the overall injury risk
Knees traveling past toes	In theory, increases injury to knee joints
Lifting too much weight	May activate GTO and muscle spindles resulting in muscles relaxing when they are not supposed to. Increase injury due poor technique and overloading muscles before they are ready.
Looking upward to the ceiling	May cause neck strain or a loss of balance
Leaning too far forward	May cause loss of balance or neck injury
Toes turning inward	May lead to knee joint injury
Locking out knees	May lead to osteoarthritis and/or other knee injuries
Knees bowing inward	May lead to knee joint injury
Uneven gripping of barbell	May lead to loss of balance
Uneven placement of barbell	May lead to loss of balance
Heels coming off the ground	May lead to loss of balance
Bar placed too low on back	May increase stress on shoulders and increase chance of barbell rolling off back
Descending too fast	Lifter misses the advantages of eccentric muscle actions
Hands not pushing up on barbell	Increases risk that bar will slide off back

Machine Seated Hamstring Curl

Primary Muscles Worked: Hamstrings (semimembranosus, semitendinosus, biceps femoris).

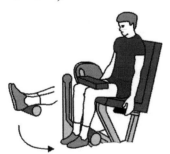

> **Quick Tip:** Align knee with rotational axis of machine.

Exercise Technique: Sit in the machine with legs over the leg pad. There should be a slight (10° to 20°) bend in the knees. If possible, adjust the lower leg pad so that it is positioned at the ankles, just above heels (at Achilles tendon). The heels should be relaxed during the movement. Check to see if the middle/rear aspect of the knees (when viewed from the side) are lined up with the axis of rotation of the machine. If not, adjust the seat. Note: the knees should be lined up with the rotational point through the full ROM. This requires testing with a light resistance first. If the machine has a thigh support pad it should be in contact with thighs (not knees). <u>Concentric phase</u>: Sitting upright in the machine with buttocks pressed into back pad and contract the abs. Now, in a controlled manner, slowly pull the legs downward halting the movement at about 90° of knee flexion. At 90 ° the lower legs will be perpendicular to the thighs. Hold contraction for a second. <u>Eccentric phase</u>: Slowly allow the legs to return to their starting position. Stop just before the weight plates of the machine touch. Repeat for the desired number of reps.

Spotting: Make sure the middle part of the knee is aligned with the machine's axis of rotation during the entire ROM. This is easiest seen when kneeling at the side of the machine. The rotation axis can sometimes be identified by a small colored dot or plastic cup that covers or highlights the axis. Make sure the toes do not rotate outward or inward as this may increase stress on the knee.

Comments & Suggestions: If the person slides down in the machine, it may be a sign of hamstring inflexibility. Some machines start the ROM with feet higher than knees which puts the knee in a hyper-extended position. This, in theory, may increase knee injuries. This machine is usually preferable to the prone version for people with heart disease and high blood pressure. In either machine, getting up too fast may case a drop in BP (orthostatic hypotension) which can cause the person to pass out.

Hamstring Curl With Stability Ball

Primary Muscles Used: Hamstrings (semimembranosus, semitendinosus, biceps femoris).

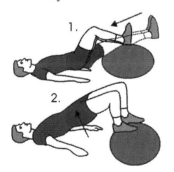

> **Quick Tip:** Keep the buttocks elevated during the exercise. Bringing the arms closer to the sides increases the difficulty.

Exercise Technique: Lie supine on the floor with a stability ball. Extend the legs and place the tops of the heels or ankles on the ball. Extend the arms out to the sides to about 45° to aid with stability. Extend the hips by pressing heels/ankles into the ball and lifting the buttocks off the floor with legs extended (maintain slight bend in the knees). This is the starting position prior to beginning the exercise. Slowly draw the ball toward you by bending at the knees. Hold for a second. Now, move the ball away by extending the legs. Stop when there is a slight bend at the knees. Repeat for the desired number of reps.

Spotting: The hips/buttocks should remain elevated and the body should not wobble while performing the exercise. The head should not come off the floor. Make sure the person is not holding their breath (Valsalva maneuver) during this exercise.

Comments & Suggestions: To perform this movement, it may be necessary to first learn with calves on ball and only raising the buttocks into air. Because this exercise uses the stability ball, more than the hamstrings are being utilized. Other muscles involved include the calves as well as the abs and back muscles. While keeping the hips elevated is important, it is not necessary to thrust the hips upward as shown in this picture. That is an advanced form of the exercise and can be something to work up to. Make sure the client can get up from the ground before using. This exercise may place stress on the cervical neck. Use with caution in those with neck problems.

Machine Prone Hamstring Curl

Primary Muscles Used: Hamstrings (semimembranosus, semitendinosus, biceps femoris).

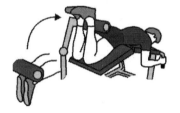

> **Quick Tip:** People with heart disease may get dizzy if they rise too fast from this machine.

Exercise Technique: Adjust the weight stack to the desired resistance. Adjust the ankle pad (if possible) so that it rests above the heels. Lay face down (prone) on the machine with the legs under the ankle pad. In this position, the knees should have a slight (10-20°) bend in them. If the machine has hand grips, grasp them lightly. The knees should be slightly off the pad. The knees should also be lined up with the rotational axis of the machine. A small, colored circular dot or plastic cup may highlight this area. The feet are relaxed. <u>Concentric phase:</u> Slowly the lift legs until a 90° bend at the knee is reached (at 90° the ankles will point straight up). <u>Eccentric phase:</u> Slowly lower to starting position, halting just before the weight stack touches the other weight plates. Do not lock out knees at the end of the eccentric phase. Repeat for the desired number of reps.

Spotting: Make sure the hips do not come off the machine as this may stress the low back. Angled benches make this less likely but it may still happen. The knees should be off the edge of the thigh pad, not pressed into the pad. There should be a slight bend at the knees when the legs are extended. The middle part of the knees should be aligned with the rotational axis of the machine. Don't let the lifter's head arch up on this exercise. Stay close to the client as they exit the machine.

Comments & Suggestions: This movement may be difficult in those with tight hamstrings than the seated hamstring curl machine. It is not necessary for the ankle pad to touch the buttocks during the concentric phase. People with heart disease and/or blood pressure issues may get dizzy if they rise too fast from this machine due a temporary drop in blood pressure (orthostatic hypotension). This may cause them to faint. For those with back problems, the seated version may be a safer alternative.

Machine Seated Leg Extension

Primary Muscles Used: Quadriceps (vastus lateralis, vastus medialis, vastus intermedius, rectus femoris.

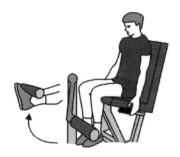

> **Quick Tip:** Align knees with rotational axis of machine.

Exercise Technique: Adjust the machine so that knees are aligned with the axis of rotation and that the leg pads are positioned above the ankles. <u>Concentric phase</u>: Slowly raise legs as high as comfortable or until soft-lock out. Do not fully lock out knees. <u>Eccentric phase</u>: Slowly lower legs to starting position halting just before the weight plates touch the weight stack. Repeat for the desired number of reps.

Spotting: Normally, the machine is adjusted so that the lifter starts when there is a 90° bend at the knees (i.e., thighs about parallel with floor) and that the knees are aligned with the rotational point of the machine. Ensure that the legs do not "lockout" at the top of the ROM. If the butt lifts off the seat during the eccentric phase, the weight is too heavy. The legs should move slowly during both concentric and eccentric phases with no quick, jerky movements. Likewise, the back should not arch up during this movement.

Comments & Suggestions: Remember that greater stresses are placed on the knee joints when the leg is extended to full (hard) lockout. Thus, the higher one lifts, in theory, the greater the risk of knee injury. As such, a soft lock out is preferred over totally locking out the knees. While this exercise is usually performed with the toes pointed straight ahead, some, research suggests that turning the toes inward (internally rotating the leg) recruits more of the vastus lateralis and vastus medialis muscles, while pointing the toes outward (externally rotating the leg) places more stress on the rectus femoris.[37] While normally performed with a 90° bend at the knee, almost any ROM is possible, if the machine has adjustable ROM limiter. The lifter's goals, strength and advice from a physical therapist (if applicable) will dictate the ROM of this exercise. Because this is a single joint exercise, it's probably wise to do it after lower body multi-joint exercises like leg presses etc. For added difficulty, perform this exercise using only one leg at a time. If knee pain is felt with this exercise, don't do it and refer to a medical professional for formal diagnosis.

Seated Inner Thigh Machine

Primary Muscles Used: Gracillis, adductor longus, adductor magnus, adductor brevis, pectineus.

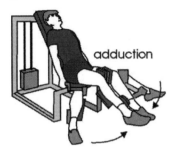

adduction

> **Quick Tip:** The inner part of the knees should be lined up with the knee pads.

Exercise Technique: If necessary, first adjust the machine so that the knee pads are close together. Sit in the machine with the inner knees aligned with the knee pads. Rest the feet on the foot supports (if applicable). Now, open the legs to a comfortable position, which for many people is when they feel a slight pull on their inner thighs. If the low back arches, the legs are open too wide. This is the starting position of the exercise. Concentric phase: Slowly close legs by pressing the knees against the knee pads until the knee pads touch each other. Hold for a second. Eccentric phase: Slowly release the tension, opening the legs to the starting position. Repeat. At the end of the set, readjust the knee pads so that the legs are close together before exiting the machine.

Spotting: The low back should not arch during the exercise. Both concentric and eccentric phases should be performed in a slow, controlled manner. If the legs open quickly while under tension, an injury may result.

Comments & Suggestions: Adduction (or AD-duction) refers to moving a body part closer (i.e., adding) to the midline of the body. While this exercise can strengthen the inner thigh muscles, it is a myth that it burns fat from the inner thighs. For most people, it's not necessary to open the legs more than about 45°. This exercise can also be performed by squeezing a stability ball between the legs. Use this exercise with caution in those who have hip replacements.

Seated Outer Thigh Machine

Primary Muscles Used: Gluteus medius, gluteus minimus, tensor fasciae latae.

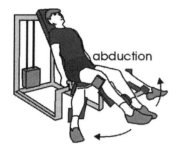

Quick Tip: The outer part of the knee should be lined up with the knee pads.

Exercise Technique: The exercise is started with the legs inside the knee pads and the legs close to each other. The knee pads should be against the outer part of the knees. In some versions, the knees are bent to 90°. Some versions also have a platform to rest the feet during the exercise. Concentric phase: Slowly press against the leg pads and open the legs to a comfortable position. Hold for a second. Eccentric phase: Slowly lower to starting position, stopping just before the weight stack touches. Repeat.

Spotting: The knees should be about parallel with the floor and in some versions, bent to about 90°. The low back should not arch during the exercise.

Comments & Suggestions: Because the hips are moving away (abducting) from the body, physical and occupational therapists often say "AB-duction" so it's not confused with "ADD-duction" described previously. It's a myth that this exercise reduces body fat (i.e., saddlebags) from the sides of the hips.

Standing Calf Raise With Dumbbell

Primary Muscles Used: Gastrocnemius.

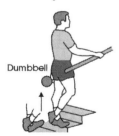

Quick Tip: Determine how low the heel can go before adding additional weight.

Exercise Technique: Obtain a dumbbell and stand on a step with the balls of the feet at the edge. The dumbbell should be held on the same side as the ankle which is to be worked. The other hand can be used for support. The foot is pointed straight ahead and there is a slight bend at the knee. Eccentric phase: Slowly lower the heel until tension is felt. Concentric phase: Rise up to the starting position or higher (i.e., plantar flexion), depending on ankle strength. Repeat.

Spotting: The knee should not be locked out. Ensure that the toes do not slide off the step during the movement. The upper body should stay neutral and neither hyperextend backward or flex forward. The head should be neutral and not turn to the sides.

Comments & Suggestions: Both the gastrocnemius and soleus are involved in plantar flexion (raising the heel upward). In this exercise, the gastrocnemius is the main muscle targeted. When seated, the soleus works more. It's safest to first determine flexibility in the calf before adding weight. The normal progression for this movement is to first perform with two feet and no added weight.

Plantar Fasciitis

Plantar fasciitis refers to inflammation of the connective tissue on the bottom of the feet and results in heel pain and stiffness that's usually felt immediately after getting out of bed or seated for a long time. It's often linked to having flat feet, tight calves and shoes that have poor arch support. The condition is often seen in those who stand for long periods of time as well as in runners, the overweight and in those who are in poor physical condition. Increasing the incline on treadmills or walking uphill may make the condition worse.. Calf flexibility is an important part of prevention and treatment. Also, using arch supports and/or icing the bottom of the foot can help the condition.

Machine Biceps Curl

Primary Muscles Used: Biceps group, brachioradialis.

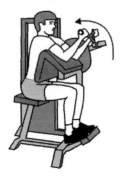

Quick Tip: Align elbows with rotation point of machine.

Exercise Technique: Adjust the seat so that the back of the arms are supported on the arm pads of the machine. The middle portion of the elbows should be aligned with the rotation point of the machine. Grasp the handles with a supinated grip. The elbows should have a slight bend in them and not be locked out. The chest should be against the chest pad of the machine. Concentric phase: Contract biceps and slowly lift until the handles are close to the shoulders or to where it feels comfortable. The wrists should not bend during the movement. <u>Eccentric phase</u>: Lower the weight in a controlled manner until there is a slight bend in elbows. Repeat for the desired number of reps.

Spotting: The elbows should be aligned with the rotational point of the machine throughout the ROM. The lifter should not rock back and forth or hunch the shoulders forward as the weight is lifted. The head does not turn to the sides.

Comments & Suggestions: Supination (palms facing up) brings the biceps into action. If the exercise is performed with a neutral grip (palms facing each other), the exercise works more of the brachialis and brachioradialis. Biceps curls may exacerbate elbow injuries (e.g., tendonitis) in those who have this injury. This is an isolation exercise that uses less muscle than a standing barbell/dumbbell curl. Use caution in those with osteoporosis; some versions may cause excessive forward trunk flexion that may increase spinal fractures.

Tennis Elbow

Tennis elbow is an overuse injury. Usually, pain is felt on the outer side (lateral side) of the elbow and results from an inflammation of a tendon. People frequently report that their elbow hurts when they pick up jars with the arm extended or when turn door knobs. Any repetitive trauma can cause tennis elbow — including doing too many sets of biceps curls. The biceps muscles tend to be overemphasized in many workout programs. Poor form (i.e., elbows moving forward during the biceps curl) can also cause this injury. Treatment usually consists of resting and icing the area followed eventually with gentle stretching and various therapeutic exercises (e.g., reverse wrist curls). For acute cases (less than 4 weeks), tennis elbow can usually be resolved in 4-6 weeks; but, if left unchecked for more than two months, the condition may become chronic and it can take up to 6 months before symptoms subside.[38] In the chronic condition, steroid injections and physical therapy or surgery may be needed.

Hammer Curl With Dumbbells

Primary Muscles Used: Brachialis, brachioradialis.

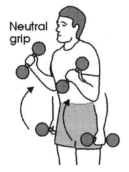

Neutral grip

Quick Tip: For added difficulty, lift dumbbells only to 90°.

Exercise Technique: This exercise can be performed standing or sitting. Grasp two equally weighted dumbbells. The dumbbells should be held in a neutral grip throughout the exercise. Concentric phase. Slowly raise dumbbells to about 90° while keeping the elbows at the sides (at 90° the forearms will be parallel, with the floor). Eccentric phase: Slowly lower to a point just before elbows lock out fully (soft lockout). Repeat for the desired number of reps.

Spotting: The trainer ensures that the elbows stay under the shoulders during the exercise. The lifter's body should not rock back and the shoulders should not shrug upward. Make certain that there is a slight bend in the knees and that the abs are contracted. The weight is lowered slowly to take advantage of the eccentric phase.

Comments & Suggestions: The neutral grip places less emphasis on the biceps group. As a result, this exercise is sometimes overlooked; however, the muscles targeted in this movement can also help with overall biceps development. This exercise might be a good alternative for those with wrist problems and may be more functional than biceps curls for people who play sports like tennis.

Triceps Pushdown

Primary Muscles Used: Triceps.

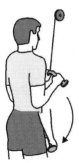

Quick Tip: Keep the elbows held to the sides of the body at all times.

Exercise Technique: Stand facing the machine and grasp the bar with a closed, pronated grip. The grip used can vary from very close to wide. The feet should be hip to shoulder width apart. The knees should be slightly flexed and there should be a slight forward lean at the hips, such that the bodyweight is aligned over the ankles. Stand close enough so that the cable hangs straight down when the exercise is performed. Pull the bar down until the arms are bent at about 90° and the elbows are tucked into the sides of the body (i.e., the forearms are parallel with floor). This is the starting point of the exercise. Concentric phase: Slowly press downward until the arms are almost straight (i.e., soft lock out). Hold for a second. Eccentric phase: Slowly release the tension, which raises the bar back up to the starting position. Repeat for the desired number of reps.

Spotting: The elbows should not move forward, away from the sides of body. This takes the stress off of the triceps. Place towels between the torso and elbows or palpate the lifter's elbows with your fingers so that the elbows remain stationary at the sides of the body. Make sure the hands are evenly spaced on the bar. The wrists should not bend and the lifter should not turn their head to the sides. The body should not rock back and forth.

Comments & Suggestions: Some people perform this exercise standing straight up at attention. At heavier resistances, this can put stress to the low back. Bending at the hips and knees reduces this risk. Some cable machines allow this exercise to be performed with the back pressed against the machine. This better stabilizes the back (good for those with back issues) yet activates the abs to a lesser degree. If a rope is used, the weight may feel heaver than with a metal bar because the rope is lighter and there is less of a counterweight effect. Because this is a single joint exercise, lifting maximum loads is not recommended.

Back Extension With Stability Ball

Primary Muscles Used: Erector spinae.

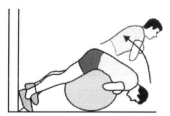

> **Quick Tip:** For added difficulty, don't anchor the feet to the wall.

Exercise Technique: Lie prone (face down) on the stability ball with the belly button positioned near or at the top of the ball. The legs are hip to shoulder width apart and extended. There should be a slight bend in the knees. The feet can be pressed against a wall or ankles held by the trainer for added stability. The hands can be at the sides, crossed over the chest or stretched out in front. Before the exercise begins, the lifter's trunk is flexed, which facilitates the upward concentric action. Concentric phase: Retract shoulder blades and slowly lift the upper body upward until it is approximately in line with the legs. Eccentric phase: Slowly lower to starting position. Repeat for the desired number of reps.

Spotting: Ensure retraction of shoulder blades throughout movement. The head should stay neutral. If stabilizing the lifter, hold at the ankles.

Comments & Suggestions: It is not necessary to hyperextend the back on this exercise. Also, it's not necessary to use added resistance (e.g., weight plates). Most people can be adequately challenged by lifting only their bodyweight. For most healthy people, 3-4 sets of 15-20 reps should be mastered before adding an external resistance. Back extensions may be inappropriate for people with some back injuries. Difficulty increases the closer the legs are to each other.

Crunch On Stability Ball

Primary Muscles Used: Rectus abdominis, internal and external obliques.

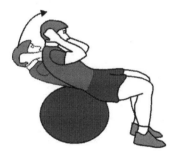

> **Quick Tip:** For added difficulty perform with one leg in the air.

Exercise Technique: Recline supine on a stability ball with feet about shoulder width apart and knees bent to about 90°. The ball should rest somewhere between the low back to middle back range, depending on fitness level and difficulty desired. Concentric phase: Contract the abs (pull the belly button inward) and slowly curl the torso upward bringing the ribs closer to the hips. Eccentric phase: Slowly lower to starting point. Repeat for the desired number of reps.

Spotting: The upper torso should curl inward and become concave as it is lifted. Clasping the hands behind the neck may increase neck strain.

Comments & Suggestions: It's not necessary to do a full sit-up. Just a slight movement is all that's needed to challenge the abs. Performed slowly, the abs should be sufficiently challenged after 12-20 reps. There are many ways to increase the difficulty of this exercise. For example, extending the arms over and behind the head or performing with one leg in the air increases difficulty. It's a myth that crunches or sit ups burn fat from the belly area. Caution: sit ups and crunches may increase fractures of the spinal cord bones in those with osteoporosis.

CHAPTER 8
Training People With Health Issues

Training People Who Have High Blood Pressure

Overview Of The Issue

➢ Also called hypertension. Abbreviated HTN. Defined as a consistent, resting BP of at least 140-90.

➢ Prehypertension is a BP of 120/80 (note. 120/80 is not called "normal" anymore).

➢ High blood pressure is a major risk factor for stroke – the 3rd leading cause of death.

➢ BP (especially systolic) tends to increase with age; Strive for a resting BP below 120/80.[39]

➢ Most cases have no known cause and are called idiopathic or primary hypertension. If the condition can be traced to another factor (obesity, etc.) it is called secondary hypertension.

➢ Not all cases of HTN can be controlled by diet and exercise alone.

➢ The following all increase risk: excess body weight, excess dietary sodium, reduced physical activity, and lack of fruits and vegetables in the diet.[39]

➢ Strength training may have a positive effect on HTN however it is less than aerobic exercise.

General Guidelines for Hypertension

➢ Lose weight if necessary. Aim for a BMI of 18.5 - 24.9.

➢ Stop smoking. Reduce saturated fat and cholesterol from diet.

➢ Sodium intake: no more than a teaspoon per day (2300 mg). Middle age people - 1500 mg might be better. The average man consumes 4000 mg sodium/day; the average woman, 3000 mg/day.

➢ Increase potassium-rich foods (fruits and vegetables). Eat according to the DASH diet. DASH stands for Dietary Approaches to Stop Hypertension. DASH emphasizes fruits, vegetables and low fat-dairy and reduces saturated fat, total fat and cholesterol intake.

➢ Alcohol. Men: No more than 2 drinks per day. Women: No more than 1 drink per day.

➢ Exercise. Aim for at least 30 minutes of exercise at least 4 days of the week.

➢ Maintain flexibility in hamstrings. Some research shows more artery damage in people with less flexible hamstrings.

Type of Exercise	Exercise Guideline	Frequency, Intensity, Time
Aerobic	Large-muscle activities, bike, treadmill, swimming etc.	RPE: 2 - 4 (0-10 scale) 30 - 60 min per day 4 - 7 day/wk Expend 700-2000 calories per week
Strength Training	Circuit training	Low resistance, higher number of reps (e.g., 15 - 20RM)

Suggestions & Comments

- ✓ If possible, take BP before and after exercise to measure how exercise alters BP.
- ✓ If client uses hypertension meds, use Borg scale or Talk Test to gauge exercise intensity.
- ✓ Don't exercise if BP is $\geq$ 200/115.
- ✓ Measure BMI and waist circumference at regular intervals .
- ✓ People must do cardio, preferably 4-7 days per week. Do not only do strength training.
- ✓ Overhead lifts should be used with caution because of Valsalva maneuver.
- ✓ Avoid static (isometric) contractions when possible. This increases BP.
- ✓ Avoid tight gripping of fitness equipment (e.g., treadmill). This increases BP.
- ✓ Avoid fast transfers from seated/supine positions to standing. They may faint.
- ✓ Lower intensity exercise is better at lowering BP than higher intensity exercise.
- ✓ HTN damages blood vessels. This increases the risk of heart attack and stroke.
- ✓ HTN can also lead to kidney failure.
- ✓ People with HTN should not lift very heavy weights. Circuit training is best for them.
- ✓ If they have prehypertension the guidelines are lifestyle changes - lose weight, lower sodium and environmental stress, exercise regularly, limit alcohol and stop smoking.
- ✓ Potassium from fruits and vegetables is better than potassium supplements.
- ✓ Consider all of their health issues when designing an exercise program.
- ✓ HTN has few symptoms that the person can feel. This is why they call it the silent killer.

Training People Who Have High Cholesterol Levels

Overview Of The Issue

- ➢ Cholesterol is a component of artery-clogging plaque.
- ➢ High cholesterol levels increase the risk for heart disease (CAD) and stroke.
- ➢ CAD risk factors: smoking, being overweight, belly fat, genetics, lack of exercise, high blood pressure, diabetes. CAD risk also increases as we grow older.
- ➢ Hypercholesterolemia refers specifically to elevated cholesterol levels (>200 mg/dl).
- ➢ Hypertriglyceridemia refers specifically to elevated triglycerides levels (>150 mg/dl).
- ➢ Hyperlipidemia refers to elevated levels of cholesterol and triglycerides.
- ➢ HDL is high density lipoprotein (good cholesterol). Transports cholesterol back to liver.
- ➢ HDL: ≥40 mg/dl is good. Strive for an HDL of 60 or better.
- ➢ LDL is low density lipoprotein (bad cholesterol). Transports cholesterol from the liver out to the cells of the body.
- ➢ LDL < 100 mg/dl is good but LDL of 70 might be better in most people.
- ➢ Breaking up exercise into smaller sessions is as good as one longer session.

Type of Exercise	Exercise Guideline	Frequency, Intensity, Time
Aerobic	Multi-joint activities: swimming, treadmill, bike, elliptical.	5-7 day per wk/ 20-60 min per session. RPE 2-4 (0-10 scale); 40-80% Karvonen HRmax
Strength Training	Circuit training or multiple set programs (begin with circuits)	Circuits: light weights (e.g., 40%-60% 1 RM) higher reps (e.g.,12-15 reps per set); multiple set programs: 2-4 sets 8-12 reps at 60-80% 1RM

Suggestions & Comments

- ✓ Losing weight often helps lower cholesterol and blood lipid levels.
- ✓ The optimal amount of exercise needed to lower lipids can vary. The main goal is to burn calories during exercise. Cardio is very efficient at burning calories.
- ✓ An HDL of 60 mg/dl or better is a "negative risk factor" for heart disease (i.e., it lowers the risk). Exercise - esp. cardio - often increases HDL.
- ✓ Aerobic exercise can increase the size of LDL - which makes the LDL not as harmful.
- ✓ If the person is using beta blockers or other medications that lower RHR, use RPE and/or Talk Test to determine how hard they are exercising.
- ✓ Determining 1RM may not be needed or advisable because of other medical issues the person may also have.
- ✓ Adding a cardio station to the strength training circuit ramps up the aerobic component of the circuit and the calories they use during exercise.

- ✓ Reduce saturated fat. Saturated fat raises cholesterol levels.
- ✓ People taking statin drugs should refrain from grapefruit and/or grapefruit juice. Some weight loss supplements may contain grapefruit.
- ✓ Dietary supplements. Some may help. Others may not. For more information read *Nutritional Supplements* available at Joe-Cannon.com

Training People Who Have Had a Heart Attack

`Overview Of The Issue

- Heart attacks result when heart muscle dies from inadequate oxygen supply. This can result when artery-clogging plaque builds up in blood vessels.
- Heart disease can lead to a heart attack and is often abbreviated as CAD by doctors.
- People who have had one heart attack, may be at risk of another. Be familiar with the signs of a heart attack and remember that high intensity exercise increases the risk.
- Doctors abbreviate heart attack as "MI" (myocardial infarction).
- Always get a written doctors note before working with people who had a heart attack (or any other significant medical disorder).

Type of Exercise	Exercise Guideline	Frequency, Intensity, Time
Aerobic	Multi-joint movements	3-4 days per week/ RPE 2-6, 20-40 min per session
Strength Training	Circuit training	2-3 days per week/ 1-3 sets of 10-15 reps
Flexibility	Improve/maintain flexibility	1-3 days per week.

Suggestions & Comments

- Doctors may quantify exercise in terms of METs. Those with low fitness levels will probably be prescribed an exercise level of 5 METs or less.
- Warm-up and cool-down. This may help stabilize heart rate before and after exercise.
- Strength training: loads lifted should be light to moderate (e.g., 10-15 reps / exercise).
- Begin with only 1 set per exercise.
- When increasing weights, 2-5 lbs for upper body exercises and 5-10 lbs for lower body may be appropriate, but can vary according to fitness level, age, and other health issues.[40]
- Rest periods between sets are generally 1.5- 2 minutes. This can vary by fitness level.[40]
- People should never hold their breath during exercise (Valsalva maneuver).
- Rising too fast from the seated, supine or prone positions may result in a drop in BP that can lead to fainting. Supervise when the person rises.
- Consider other health issues when developing the exercise program.
- If the person takes beta blockers or other medications that slow HR, use RPE Scale.
- People who complain of pain in their ankles or legs upon walking, only to have it subside after stopping the activity, may have peripheral artery disease (abbreviated as PAD or PVD). Stationary bicycle or upper body aerobic exercise (e.g., UBE) may be good options for them.

- ✓ Depression may occur after a heart attack. Point out progress made and goals achieved to foster continued exercise participation.
- ✓ Try to improve activities of daily living (ADLs) if necessary

Training People With Diabetes

Overview Of The Issue

➤ Insulin helps the body use sugar (glucose). Insulin is made in the beta cells of the pancreas.

➤ There are two main types of diabetes. In type I diabetes, the person does not make insulin (or make enough) and must inject insulin. In type II diabetes, the person makes insulin but can't use it. Most cases of diabetes are type II. All type I diabetics inject insulin. Type II diabetics may also inject insulin as their disease progresses.

➤ Normal blood sugar is <100 mg/dl.

➤ Type I diabetes is caused by an autoimmune disorder. The immune system attacks the beta cells which make insulin. This decreases/shuts down insulin production.

➤ Type II diabetes appears to result from problems with insulin receptors. Lack of insulin receptors reduces the ability of insulin to work. Without insulin receptors the body becomes "insulin resistant." They make insulin but are resistant to its effects.

➤ Metabolic Syndrome. A group of conditions that increase risk for type II diabetes. Symptoms include abdominal obesity, reduced HDL, increased LDL and triglycerides, insulin resistance and increased blood pressure. Elevated CRP levels sometimes also noted. Exercise can improve metabolic syndrome.

➤ Gestational diabetes. Diabetes that occurs during pregnancy. This increases the risk of future type II diabetes in the mother.

➤ Hemoglobin A1c: A marker of blood sugar levels over the last 3 months. Normal: < 6

➤ Diabetes may be accompanied by heart disease, vision problems, kidney problems, balance problems and hypertension, to name a few. Many people die from the complications of diabetes.

➤ Hypoglycemia. Low blood sugar. Signs can include rapid heart rate, sweating, anxiety, tremors, mental confusion and ultimately loss of consciousness.

➤ Ketosis. Abnormal elevation in ketones. Results from burning fat without the presence of carbs (glucose). Ketosis upsets acid/base balance of body. If not treated, can lead to death.

Type of Exercise	Exercise Guideline	Frequency, Intensity, Time
Aerobic	Multi-joint activities, treadmill, swimming, bike etc.	50%-90% HR max, 20-60 min per session. Most days of week.
Strength training	Machines, free weights or combination.	Improve strength and muscle endurance. Use caution with high intensity exercise.

Suggestions & Comments

✓ Diabetes may reduce flexibility in the hands, fingers and shoulders. Maintain flexibility.

- ✓ Don't exercise if blood sugar is > 250 mg/dl.
- ✓ Signs of low blood sugar (hypoglycemia): shaking, dizziness, rapid heart rate, hunger, blurry vision, headache, fatigue, weakness or irritability, sweating.
- ✓ If diabetic becomes unconscious, it's safest to give sugar (carbs). If hypoglycemia is the reason the person passed out and insulin is administered, blood sugar will go even lower – which can be fatal.
- ✓ Signs of ketosis: dry mouth; rapid, deep breathing, feeling very tired and being very thirsty. Fruity smelling breath, confusion, nausea and/or vomiting, coma.
- ✓ Person should carry carbohydrates with them or they should easily be accessed.
- ✓ Client should be aware of the different types of insulin and when they are most effective at lowering blood sugar and avoid workouts when the insulin they are using is most effective.
- ✓ Avoid exercising the area of the body that was injected with insulin.
- ✓ Holding breath during strength training may damage already weakened blood vessels.
- ✓ Measure blood sugar before and after exercise – especially when starting a new program.
- ✓ Balance and vision problems are common. Stay with client at all times.
- ✓ Loss of feeling in the feet (neuropathy) can lead to poor balance. Because of this, injuries to the feet (blisters, broken bones etc.) may not be noticed.
- ✓ Remember that higher intensities of exercise may raise blood sugar.

Training People Who Have Asthma

Overview Of The Issue

➢ Symptoms of asthma include tightness or pain in the chest, coughing and shortness of breath. Wheezing can sometimes be heard when the person breathes.

➢ Both genetics and environmental stress (dust etc.) can cause asthma symptoms.

➢ Exercise may exacerbate asthma symptoms (exercise-induced asthma) in some people but long term exercise can help asthma also.

➢ There is no proof that people with asthma should avoid exercise.

➢ Symptoms often appear at exercise intensities of 75% max HR or higher. Lower intensities may provoke asthma symptoms also.

➢ Exercising in cold temperatures can bring about an asthmatic attack. Environmental /airborne pollutants (exhaust fumes, perfume etc.) can also trigger attacks.

➢ Risk factors can include, genetics, exposure to second hand smoke, living in areas with a lot of pollution, being overweight and having frequent infections as a child.

Exercise Guidelines

Type of Exercise	Exercise Guideline	Frequency, Intensity, Time
Aerobic Exercise	Multi-joint activities	3-5 days/wk; RPE 1-4; at least 30 min.
Strength Training	Circuit training	Light resistance, higher reps; 2-3 days per week

Suggestions & Comments

✓ Person should have their inhaler with them and use it according to their doctors instructions.

✓ Personal trainers: avoid cologne / perfume. This may trigger an asthma attack.

✓ Warming up prior to aerobic exercise may help reduce an asthma attack.

✓ Clients may be very deconditioned. Progress slowly. Increase the length of time they exercise before increasing the intensity of exercise.

✓ Allow approximately 1.5 months for the person to become accustomed to exercise and get used to how they feel during exercise. This can help reduce asthma attacks.

✓ Monitor exercise exertion with Borg Scale rather than heart rate.

✓ Older clients may also have CAD, osteoporosis etc. Consider these also when designing the exercise program.

✓ Long periods of aerobic exercise tends to cause more asthma attacks than shorter periods.

✓ If working out in the cold, wear a mask to cover mouth and nose. This will help warm air and reduce flare-ups. Avoid exercise when there is a lot of pollen or pollution in the air.

Training People Who Have Arthritis

Overview of the Issue

➢ The two most common forms of arthritis are osteoarthritis (OA or DJD) and rheumatoid arthritis (RA).

➢ OA results from a wearing away of the joint cartilage. Can be caused by injury, ballistic sports participation or being overweight/obese. Genetics is also possible.

➢ RA is thought to result from an autoimmune disorder. The immune system disrupts joint integrity, causing inflammation. Eventually this destroys joint cartilage and bones.

➢ Exercise can help reduce arthritis pain.

Exercise Guidelines

Type of Exercise	Exercise Guideline	Frequency, Intensity, time
Aerobic	Mulit-joint movements. Pool exercise is optimal for some	3-5 days per wk/ RPE 2-6 / 5-30 min per day
Strength Training	Circuit training	2-3 days per week/ 2-12 reps. Intensity varies with pain levels.

Suggestions & Comments

✓ Warm up before exercise.

✓ Start at a low intensity. Increase the time they exercise before increasing the intensity.

✓ Strength training: machines are often easier to use than free weights.

✓ If needed, break exercise up into several small sessions.

✓ Chair-based exercise may be needed for those with poor balance/functional ability.

✓ Activities that focus on balance, walking and ADLs can help improve quality of life.

✓ Those with RA may have more stiffness in the morning. This may make early workouts more difficult.

✓ If possible, they should move a little even when their symptoms feel worse. This will help maintain strength, reduce pain, and help cardiovascular function.

✓ Isometric exercises may be needed before dynamic movements in the very deconditioned.

✓ Avoid high repetition, high impact activities and those that use high levels of resistance.

✓ Pool exercise can help improve aerobic endurance if land exercise is not possible.

✓ People often confuse osteoarthritis with osteoporosis. They are not the same.

✓ Consider all other conditions they have when designing an exercise program.

✓ Maintaining flexibility is good but too much flexibility may make their joints unstable.

Training People Who Have Fibromyalgia

Overview of the Issue

➢ Fibromyalgia is a condition marked by widespread pain and stiffness that's felt in the muscles, ligaments and tendons. Pain is felt at specific areas (tender points).

➢ Tender points include the upper chest, back of the head, upper back, neck, elbows, hips and knees. Fatigue and depression are also common as is numbness in hands and/or feet.

➢ To be diagnosed: 1.) Must be in pain for at least 3 months and 2.) Pain must be specific to at least 11 of the 18 known tender points. All other causes of symptoms must be ruled out also.

➢ Pain varies according to emotions, stress, exercise, lack of sleep.

➢ People may not sleep well. Lack of quality sleep increases feelings of pain/fatigue.

➢ Many are sensitive to cold, touch and bright lights. Migraine headaches may also occur.

➢ Some research suggests there may be a relationship to a hypersensitivity of nerves which conduct feelings of pain in response to stimuli that normally isn't painful.

➢ Some may have elevations in a chemical called substance P which signals feelings of pain.

➢ Classified as a form of arthritis. The cause of fibromyalgia is unknown.

Exercise Guidelines

Type of Exercise	Exercise Guideline	Frequency, Intensity, Time
Aerobic	Use large muscle groups. Pool exercise may be needed for some.	2-3 days per week, Low intensity. Focus on time of exercise rather than intensity; 20-40 min per day.
Strength training	Use light resistance	Light resistances. Increasing reps performed is safer than increasing resistances used.
Flexibility	Stretch before, during, after exercise	Stretch to mild discomfort only. Never stretch to pain.

Suggestions & Comments

✓ Eccentric exercises (negatives) may aggravate fibromyalgia.

✓ Pool exercise can help. This also reduces eccentric the nature of resistance exercise.

✓ Many have poor balance. Monitor closely.

✓ Many with fibromyalgia have poor aerobic capacity.

✓ If doing multiple set programs, longer rest periods between sets may be needed.

✓ Don't exercise until fatigue sets in. Too much exercise makes symptoms worse.

✓ Pain experienced can change each day. This can reduce loads lifted. Don't focus on intensity of exercise. Have them exercise longer if possible rather than harder.

✓ Fibromyalgia is not the same chronic fatigue syndrome.

✓ Because it limits movement, fibromyalgia may increase the risk of other conditions (e.g. type II diabetes).

✓ People may need more than 48 hrs to recover from exercise, especially in the beginning.

✓ Point out the goals they achieved and progress they make. They may not be aware of this.

✓ The main goals are to help them feel better, improve exercise tolerance and improve ADLs.

Training People Who Have Chronic Fatigue Syndrome

Overview of the Issue

- CFS is defined as having long term, fatigue of unknown origin. Rest does not make it better.
- Some symptoms include having sore throats, poor concentration/short term memory, headaches, joint pain and exaggerated fatigue several days after exercise.
- Some people confuse CFS with fibromyalgia. They are not the same.

Exercise Guidelines

Type of Exercise	Exercise Guideline	Frequency, Intensity, Time
Aerobic Exercise	Pool, treadmill, bike elliptical. Use what they like doing.	10-30 minutes 2-4 days per week
Strength Training	Multi-joint activities	Light weight, RPE 1-3
Flexibility	Static stretching	Gentle stretch. Hold 2-15 seconds. Repeat if needed.

Suggestions & Comments

- Focus on helping them feel better and maintaining current levels of fitness. For the first few months, don't worry about improvements in strength or endurance.
- Use RPE scale to determine exercise intensity. Keep RPE very light (~1) at first.
- DOMS will make them feel worse. Minimize DOMS at all costs. Advise people that they may feel increased fatigue and a little DOMS in the beginning.
- People may need more than 48 hrs to recover from exercise, especially in the beginning.
- Point out the goals they achieved and progress they make.
- Because of a lack of understanding about how to treat CFS, people may try various alternative medicine practices, including dietary supplements. Be a good resource to help dispel myths and sort fact from fiction.

Training People Who Have HIV

Overview of the Issue

- ➤ HIV is the virus that causes AIDS.
- ➤ HIV and AIDS are not the same. AIDS is the disease caused by HIV infection.
- ➤ People with HIV can exercise if their doctor says it's ok.
- ➤ Some with HIV may be very deconditioned. Begin exercise at a low level.
- ➤ People with HIV may progress in fitness at slower rates than others.

Exercise Guidelines

Type of Exercise	Exercise Guideline	Frequency, Intensity, Time
Aerobic Exercise	Maintain /improve aerobic endurance	3-4 days per week; 40%-60% Karvonen HR; 30-60 min per day
Strength Training	Maintain/improve muscle strength	2-3 sets 8-10 reps

Suggestions & Comments

- ✓ Obtain note from physician prior to training. If possible, speak to their health care provider to determine if there are any restrictions for exercise.
- ✓ Record body weight, circumferences and BMI regularly. Take note of any decreases.
- ✓ AIDS can lead to muscle and bone loss which can result in decreases in strength and aerobic capacity.
- ✓ Strength training: focus on large muscle groups. 60% 1RM may be appropriate for some but this can vary according to their fitness level. Some need lighter resistances.
- ✓ Avoid training to exhaustion. Exhaustive exercise weakens the immune system. Do not push clients beyond their ability.
- ✓ Germs can reside on fitness equipment in the gym. If possible disinfect equipment before the client uses it. This may help reduce infections.
- ✓ Balance training can help. As HIV progresses it may reduce balance and coordination.
- ✓ It is highly unlikely that fitness trainers will get HIV from training someone who has the virus. Trainers should avoid contact with bodily fluids. If coming in contact with body fluids, wear gloves.
- ✓ Frequent exercise modifications may be needed if HIV progresses.
- ✓ Trainers should not discuss personal and private medical issues with others in a way that identifies the client. This is true for all health issues, not just HIV.
- ✓ Clients should consult their physician before taking immune boosting supplements.

Training People Who Have Osteoporosis

Overview of the Issue

➢ Mostly affects postmenopausal women. It usually occurs between 50-70 years of age. In men, osteoporosis becomes significant after age 70.

➢ Relevant bone cells: osteoblasts are bone-making cells. Osteocytes are mature bone cells. Osteoclasts are bone-eating cells.

➢ Estrogen causes death to osteoclasts and extends life of osteoblasts. After menopause, estrogen decreases and osteoclast activity ramps up, accelerating bone loss.

➢ By the 40s some bone loss has probably occurred in most people. Building strong bones in youth reduces prevalence in old age. Poor/inadequate nutrition can promote osteoporosis at younger ages.

➢ Osteoporosis risk factors: gender, amenorrhea, low BMI, ethnicity, genetics, age, thin bones and various lifestyle factors.

➢ Life style factors: lack of calcium and vitamin D, lack of proper exercise, smoking, excess alcohol.

➢ Osteopenia: pre-osteoporosis. Significant bone loss has occurred but not yet considered osteoporosis. May progress to osteoporosis unless intervention occurs.

Exercise Guidelines

Type of Exercise	Exercise Guideline	Frequency, Intensity, Time
Aerobic	Work large muscle groups	40-70% maximum heart rate. 30-60 minutes per day, most days of the week
Strength training	Large muscle groups; machines, free weights are appropriate	2-3 sets of 75% 1RM or 3 sets 8-10 RM. 2-3 days per week

Suggestions & Comments

✓ Beginners: low resistances/high reps (12-20 reps) for first few months.

✓ Some will have poor/reduced aerobic capacity because their lungs can't expand as much.

✓ Their center of gravity may change. This contributes to poor balance.

✓ Train balance as well as strength and aerobic ability.

✓ Weight bearing activity is not always strength training. Weight bearing only occurs when standing/walking.

✓ Stay with people when they are on the treadmill to reduce fall risk.

✓ Avoid crunches /sit ups. They may increase spinal cord fractures.

✓ Avoid exercises that involve twisting of the spine.

✓ Use lighter loads for single joint exercises to reduce injuries.

✓ Calcium from food appears better at building bones than calcium supplements.

✓ Calcium supplements: calcium carbonate and calcium citrate are preferred.

✓ Calcium RDA: 1200-1500 mg/day.

✓ Vitamin D RDA: 400-1000 IU/day.

✓ Consider other syndromes the person may have when prescribing exercise.

✓ Many people confuse osteoporoses with osteoarthritis.

Training Older Adults

Overview of the Issue

- Exercise can help reduce the risk of many diseases the plague older adults.
- Less than 10% of people over the age of 65 lift weights.
- The older people get, the less likely they are to strength train.
- Older adults who are frail or who cannot perform one or more ADLs have a greater chance of living in a nursing home one day.
- Many have sarcopenia as well as osteoporosis, osteoarthritis, heart disease and diabetes.

Type of Exercise	Exercise Guideline	Frequency, Intensity, time
Aerobic	Start at low intensity. Increase time of exercise before intensity.	3-5 days/week, low intensity as tolerated, 5-60 min per day
Strength Training	Start at low intensity	2-3 days/week, intensity varies according to fitness level

Suggestions & Comments

- The Talk Test and/or RPE scale are usually better/easier than target heart rate for determining exercise intensity.
- Older adults may take longer to recuperate between sets. 2-5 minutes may be needed.
- Always warm up and cool down.
- Remind older adults to hydrate. Their thirst sensation may be dulled.
- Remind older adults to breath when lifting weights. This reduces the Valsalva maneuver.
- Develop functional strength (i.e. standing up) and improve ADLs where needed.
- Balance training may reduce the risk of falls.
- Supervise when people are on the treadmill to reduce fall risk.
- Fast transfers to standing may cause a drop in blood pressure causing them to faint.
- If walking is not possible, consider pool or chair-based exercise programs.
- Train tibialis anterior muscles to improve walking and reduce fall risk.
- Avoid crunches /sit ups/spinal flexion in those with osteoporosis.
- Avoid seated preacher curl machines (that cause spinal flexion) in those with osteoporosis.
- Avoid static/isometric contractions. This may raise blood pressure too much especially when combined with Valsalva maneuver.
- Use language the person can understand. Demonstrate exercises before they perform them.
- Older adults may have multiple medical issues. Consider all of them when designing an exercise program.

Training Children & Adolescents

Overview of the Issue

- Prepubescent children sweat less than adults and take longer to sweat. This makes them more vulnerable to overheating.
- If exercising in the heat, slowly introduce exercise and give frequent hydration breaks.
- Encourage children to drink fluids. They may not want to.
- Properly designed and supervised strength training programs do not appear to stunt the growth of children. Unsupervised or poorly made programs may do this however.
- Before puberty, children gain strength mainly through neurological changes, not muscle hypertrophy.

Type of Exercise	Exercise Guideline	Frequency Intensity Time
Aerobic Exercise	Games, bike, treadmill. Actives they enjoy	20-60 min /day most days of the week. Exercise does not all have to be at the same time.
Strength Training	Machines, free weights, exercise tubing, soup cans, etc.	2-3 day/wk. resistance 12-20 reps. Emphasize technique over weight lifted.

Suggestions & Comments

- ✓ The exercise program should include aerobic and strength training as well as flexibility.
- ✓ Exercise program should address any specific needs the parents of the child has.
- ✓ With children, focus on exercise form /technique rather than the amount of weight lifted.
- ✓ With children, it's not necessary to determine RM values.
- ✓ Be approachable to children and speak in language that they can understand.
- ✓ Watch cartoons and TV shows that are popular with children. This helps you relate to them.
- ✓ Young children may be shy around strangers. Be encouraging and supportive.
- ✓ With children, RPE appears better than heart rate for monitoring exercise intensity. If RPE does not work well, use the Talk Test.
- ✓ Make exercise fun. Exercise programs for children do not have to be as specific as for adults.
- ✓ Children do not often exercise aerobically for long periods of time (e.g. 30 min). Rather, they do intervals, i.e. they run a short distance. Then walk a little. Then run again.
- ✓ Adolescents are still growing. As such they may be at increased risk of fractures. This risk is increased when lifting very heavy weights.
- ✓ Adolescents often have many questions about muscle building and weight loss supplements. Be able to educate them -and their parents - about fact vs. fiction.

Glossary

Abduction. Also called Ab-duction. To move a body part away from the body.

Adduction. Also called AD-duction.. To move a body part closer to the body.

ADL. Activity of daily living. Everyday tasks. Walking up stairs, carrying groceries are examples. of ADLs.

Aerobic Exercise. Activity that uses oxygen to generate energy. Cardiovascular exercise.

Anaerobic Exercise. Activity that does not require oxygen to make energy.

Antagonist Muscle. A muscle or muscles that oppose the prime mover. The triceps are antagonistic to the biceps during the biceps curl.

ATP. Adenosine Triphosphate. The body's main energy molecule.

Atrophy. The loss of fitness.

BIA. Bioelectric impedance analysis. A method of measuring body fat.

Bod Pod. A method of measuring body fat.

bpm. beats per minute.

BMD. Bone mineral density.

BMI. Body mass index.

BMR. Basal Metabolic Rate. The lowest metabolism possible.

Borg Scale. Also called RPE scale. A 0-10 scale used to estimate exercise intensity.

Concentric Muscle Action. In weightlifting, it's when the weight is lifted.

CPT. Certified Personal Trainer. Does not mean the same as "PT" (physical therapist)

CRP. C-reactive protein. marker of inflammation. implicated in heart disease.

Creatine Phosphate. Anaerobic energy molecule that helps regenerate ATP very fast.

Deconditioned. Not used to exercise.

DOMS. Delayed Onset Muscle Soreness.

Diastolic Blood Pressure. Pressure in the CV system when the heart is filling with blood.

Eccentric Muscle Action. In weightlifting, it's where the weight is lowered. Also called "negatives".

Ejection Fraction. The percentage of blood ejected from the heart with each heart beat.

Fast twitch muscle fiber. Type II muscle fiber.

FITT Principle. Frequency, Intensity, Time and Type of exercise.

Glucose. Blood sugar.

Glycogen. Storage form of glucose in the body.

Glycolysis. Anaerobic energy system. Uses glucose to make energy (ATP).

GTO. Golgi tendon organ. relaxes muscle if it "thinks" too much weight is being lifted.

HDL. High density lipoprotein. Also called "good" cholesterol.

Hemoglobin A1c. HbA1c. Measures long term blood sugar levels and progression of diabetes.

HR. abbreviation for Heart Rate. Maximum heart rate is Max HR or HRmax.

Hypertension. Abbreviated as HTN. High blood pressure.

Hypertrophy. An increase in size.

Hyperplasia. An increase in cell number.

Hypoglycemia. Low blood sugar.

Idiopathic. Unknown cause.

Isotonic Muscle Action. Composed to two phases called concentric and eccentric. AKA dynamic.

Krebs Cycle. Aerobic energy system. Breaks down of fat for energy.

Lactic acid. Also called lactate. A byproduct that causes the burning sensation during exercise.

LDL. Low density lipoprotein. The so-called "bad" cholesterol.

Macronutrient. Proteins, fats and carbohydrates are the macronutrients.

MET. Metabolic equivalents. METs are another way to measure exercise intensity.

Metabolic Syndrome. Several symptoms that occur together that increase risk of type II diabetes.

M.I. Heart attack.

Multi Joint Exercise. An exercise that uses many muscles simultaneously.

Neutral grip. In weight lifting, when the hands are facing each other

Obese. A BMI greater than 30 is considered obese.

Osteoporosis. A disease where bones become brittle and break easily.

Periodization. The exercise program is divided into different cycles or phases.

Prehypertension. A consistent, resting blood pressure that's 120/80 mm Hg – 139/89 mm Hg.

Prime Mover. Also called the agonist. The muscle primary responsible for the movement.

Prone. Position where the person is on his/her stomach or when the hands are facing downward.

Rhabdomyolysis. Destruction of muscle fibers. Can be caused by too much exercise.

RHR. Resting heart rate.

RICE. In first aid, Rest, Ice, Compression, Elevation

RM. Repetition Maximum.

ROM. Range of motion

RPE Scale. Ratings of Perceived Exertion Scale. The Borg Scale.

Sarcopenia. Loss of muscle during the aging process.

Sedentary. Does not exercise regularly

Single-Joint Exercise. Uses less muscle. Ex. biceps curl.

Slow twitch muscle. also called Type I muscle fibers

Soft-Lock Out. When the joint is not totally locked out.

Sticking Point. The most difficult part of a weight lifting exercise.

Supine. When the person is lying on the back or when the palms of the hands are facing upward.

Synergist Muscle. A helper /stabilizer muscle.

Systolic Blood Pressure. The blood pressure when the heart is in its pumping blood.

THR. Target Heart Rate.

Triglyceride. Another name for fat.

Type I Muscle Fibers. Slow twitch muscle fibers.

Type II Muscle Fibers. Fast twitch muscle fibers.

Valsalva Maneuver. Holding the breath during exercise. This increases blood pressure.

VO$_2$. The *volume of oxygen* used to make energy aerobically. Used as a measure of exercise intensity.

Volume. In weight lifting, defined as the weight x reps x sets.

References

1. McArdle, W. D., Katch, F. I., Katch, V. L. (1999). Sport & Exercise Nutrition. Lippincott, Williams & Wilkins.

2. Fleck SJ et al. (2003). Designing Resistance Training Programs, 3rd edition. Human Kinetics

3. Cerny FT and Burton HW (2001). Exercise Physiology for Health Car Professionals. Human Kinetics.

4. Bachle TR and Earle RW (2000). Essentials of Strength Training and Conditioning, 2nd edt. Human Kinetics.

5. Komi PV (1992). Strength and Power in Sport. Blackwell.

6. Brown LE (2007). Strength Training. National Strength & Conditioning Association. Human Kinetics.

7. Newham, et al. (1987). Repeated high - Force Eccentric Exercise: Effects on Muscle Pain and Damage. Journal of Applied Physiology 63,41381-1386.

8. No authors. Your high blood pressure questions answered – blood pressure and exercise. American Heart Association www.americanheart.org/presenter.jhtml?identifier=3034814 (accessed 3/8/07).

9. Hough, T. (1902). Ergographic studies in muscular soreness. American Journal of Physiology 7, 76-92.

10. Friden J & Lieber RJ (1992). Structural and mechanical basis of exercise- induced muscle injury. Medicine and Science in Sport and Exercise 24,5 521-530.

11. Sayers P (1999). The etiology of exercise induced muscle damage. Canadian Journal of Applied Physiology. 24,3,234-248

12. Smith, L et al. (1993). The effects of static and ballistic stretching on delayed onset muscle soreness and creatine kinase. Research Quarterly for Exercise and Sport, 64,1, 103 - 107.

13. Cannon, J (2006). Nutritional Supplements: What Works and Why. A Review from A to Zinc and Beyond. Available at www.joe-cannon.com.

14. Schwane JA & Armstrong RB (1983). Effects of training on skeletal muscle injury form downhill running in rats. Journal of Applied Physiology 55,3, 969- 975.

15. Smith, LL (1991). Acute inflammation: the underlying mechanism in delayed onset muscle soreness? Medicine and Science in Sport and Exercise 23,5 543 - 551.

16. No authors. Exertional Rhabdomyolysis and Acute Renal Impairment -New York City and Massachusetts, 1988. Morbidity and Mortality Weekly Report. October 26, 1990, 39,42,751-756.

17. Springer BL et al. (2003). Two cases of exertional rhabdomyolysis precipitated by personal trainers. Medicine and Science in sports and exercise,35, 9,1499-1502.

18. Brudvig TJ (2007). Identification of the signs and symptoms of acute exertional rhabdomyolysis in athletes: a guide for the practitioner. Strength and Conditioning Journal, 29,1,10-14.

19. Springer BL et al. (2003). Two cases of exertional rhabdomyolysis precipitated by personal trainers. Medicine and Science in sports and exercise,35, 9,1499-1502.

20. Kao PF et al. (2004). Rectus abdominis rhabdomyolysis after sit ups: unexpected detection by bone scan. British Journal of Sports Medicine, 32,3,253-254.

21. Kohut M, et al. (2002). Exercise and psychosocial factors modulate immunity to influenza vaccine in elderly individuals. Journal of Gerontology, 57A(9): M557–M562.

22. Peters, R.K., Bateman, E.D. (1983). Ultramarathon running an upper respiratory track infections. South African Medical Journal, 64, 582-584.

23. Fox E, Bowers R and Foss M (1993). The Physiological Basis for Exercise and Sport. Fifth edition. Brown & Benchmark

24. No author. What are high blood pressure and prehypertension? National Heart Lung Blood Institute. http://www.nhlbi.nih.gov/hbp/hbp/whathbp.htm (accessed 8/21/07).

25. ACSM's Guidelines for Exercise Testing and Prescription, 6th edition. Lippincott Williams & Williams.

26. Graves JE et al. (1988). Effects of reduced training frequency on muscular strength. International Journal of Sports Medicine 9,316-319.

27. Gettman LR et a (1981). Circuit weight training: a critical review of its physiological benefits. The physician and Sports Medicine, 9,44-60

28. Gotshalk, LA et al. (2004). Cardiovascular responses to a high-volume continuous circuit resistance training protocol. Journal of Strength and Conditioning Research, 18,4 760-764.

29. Calder AW et al. (1994). Comparison of whole and split weight raining routines in young women. Canadian Journal of Applies Physiology, 19,2,185-199.

30. Higbie EJ et al. (1996). Effect of concentric and eccentric training on muscle strength cross sectional area and neural activation. Journal of Applied Physiology, 812173-2181.

31. Hunter GR et al. (2003). Comparison of metabolic and heart rate responses to super slow vs. traditional resistance training. Journal of Strength and Conditioning Specialists, 17,1,76-81.

32. Keeler LK et al. (2001). Early phase adaptations of training speed vs. superslow resistance training on strength and aerobic capacity in sedentary individuals. Journal of Strength and Conditioning Research, 15, 309-314.

33. National Heart, Lung, and Blood Institute, National Institutes of Health (2000). The Practical Guide: Identification, Evaluation, and Treatment of Overweight and Obesity in Adults (NIH Publication No. 00-4084). www.nhlbi.nih.gov/guidelines/obesity/prctgd_c.pdf (accessed 4/7/08).

34. Green C M et al. (2007). Effect of grip width on bench press on bench press performance and risk of injury. Strength and Conditioning Journal, 29,5,10-14.

35. Gerben C (2007). Deep venous thrombosis, upper extremity. E Medicine. ww.emedicine.com/radio/topic774.htm (accessed 3/15/08).

36. Crate T (June 1997). Analysis of the lat pull down. Strength and Conditioning, 76.

37. Stoutenberg M et al. (2006). Impact of foot position on electromyographical activity of the superficial quadriceps muscle during leg extension. Journal of Strength and Conditioning Research, 19,4, 931-938.

38. Safran M et al. Instructions for Sports Medicine Patients. Elsevier Publishers.

39. Seventh report of the Joint National Committee on Prevention, Detection, Evaluation and Treatment of High Blood Pressure. US department of health and human services. www.nhlbi.nih.gov/guidelines/hypertension/jnc7full.htm (accessed 4/17/08).

40. Ehlke K (2006). Resistance exercise for post myocardial infarction patients: current guidelines and future considerations, Journal of Strength and Conditioning, 28,6, 56-62.

Index

About Joe Cannon

Joe Cannon holds an MS degree in Exercise Science and a BS degree in Chemistry & Biology. He is a self-employed personal trainer, consultant, freelance writer and blogger. He has been on the AAAI/ISMA educational faculty for over 10 years, lecturing about personal training - healthy and not so healthy people - sports nutrition, wellness and dietary supplements.

He is doubly certified by the National Strength & Conditioning Association (NSCA) as both a Certified Strength and Conditioning Specialist (CSCS) and as a Personal Trainer (NSCA-CPT).

Joe is the author of several books including

- Personal Fitness Training Beyond The Basics
- Nutritional Supplements What Works and Why
- The Personal Trainers Big Book of Questions & Answers
- Personal Trainer Practice Test
- Nutrition Essentials

He has written for several online and print publications including Fitness Management, Today's Dietitian and the Journal of Strength and Conditioning to name a few.

For Joe's dietary supplement reviews visit www.Supplement-Geek.com

To receive Joe's Personal Trainer Email Newsletter or contact Joe directly, visit his website www.Joe-Cannon.com

Made in the USA
Lexington, KY
09 August 2015